BLOOD, SWEAT AND TEA

BLOOD, SWEAT AND TEA

Real-life Adventures in an Inner-City Ambulance

Tom Reynolds

WINDSOR
PARAGON

First published 2006
by The Friday Project
This Large Print edition published 2010
by BBC Audiobooks Ltd
by arrangement with
HarperCollins*Publishers*

Hardcover ISBN: 978 1 408 46066 5
Softcover   ISBN: 978 1 408 46067 2

British Library Cataloguing in Publication Data available

Printed and bound in Great Britain by CPI Antony
Rowe, Chippenham and Eastbourne

Dedicated to my mum and brother, who have had to put up with me all these years. Also to the patients who have given me such pleasure and writing material. Finally to my workmates in the London Ambulance Service, who are the best bunch of under-appreciated workers I've ever had the privilege to know.

🚑 PROLOGUE: TOO YOUNG

Yesterday started well, we had the only new 'yellow' vehicle on the complex, and it really is an improvement on the old motors. But then we got a job that should have been routine, but unfortunately was not.

We were given a '34-year-old male, seizure' at a nearby football pitch in the middle of a park. Also leaving from our station was the FRU (a fast car designed to get to a scene before the ambulance). As we had a new motor, we were able to keep up with the FRU.

Arriving at the top of the street, we were met and directed by some of the patient's football team-mates. Unfortunately, the patient was 200 yards into the park, and there was no way we were going to get the ambulance onto the field—the council had built a little moat around the park to stop joyriders tearing up the grass in their stolen cars.

The FRU paramedic had reached the patient first and I ran across the field to get to the patient as the paramedic looked worried, and this isn't someone who normally worries.

As I reached the patient, carrying the scoop which we would use to move him, the paramedic asked me if I thought the patient was breathing.

The patient was Nigerian, and it is not racist to say that sometimes detecting signs of life on a black person is harder than if the patient is Caucasian. White people tend to look dead; black people often just look unconscious. Also, a windy playing field at dusk is not the ideal circumstance to assess a patient.

'He's not breathing' I told the paramedic, just as my crewmate reached us. 'Shit' replied the paramedic, 'I left the FR2 [An FR2 is a defibrillation machine, which is used to shock a heart back into a normal rhythm: in the UK emergency medical technicians (EMTs) are allowed to use this piece of equipment, and rapid defib' shocks are essential in certain forms of cardiac arrest] in my car'.

I had to run 200 yards back to our ambulance to get this, now vital, piece of kit.

On my return my colleagues had started to 'bag' the patient (this means using equipment to 'breathe for' the patient and performing cardiopulmonary resuscitation, or CPR), which is the procedure to keep blood flowing around the body in the absence of a pulse. Attaching the defib' pads I saw that the patient was in 'fine VF' (ventricular fibrillation)—this is a heart rhythm which means the heart is 'quivering' rather than pumping blood around the body to the brain and other vital organs. Technically, the patient is dead and without immediate treatment, they will remain dead.

We 'shocked' the patient once and his heart rhythm changed. It changed to asystole (this means that the heart is not moving at all, and it is much more difficult to restore life to the patient with this form of rhythm). We decided to 'scoop and run' to the nearest hospital. The paramedic secured the patient's airway by passing a tube down the windpipe, and we got the patient onto the scoop, all the time continuing the CPR and giving

2

potentially lifesaving drugs. We then carried him, with the help of his team-mates, to the ambulance and rushed him to hospital.

Unfortunately, the patient never regained consciousness, and died in the resuscitation room.

Thirty-four years old, normally fit and healthy—and he drops dead on a football pitch. Despite our best efforts there was nothing more we could have done for him; the treatment went according to plan and the resuscitation attempt went smoothly. This was a 'proper' job, but one job we would have happily done without.

🚑 WHY WON'T THEY LET ME DO THIS?

Here is a moan about something that I am not allowed to do. I'm not allowed to run people over in my job. I could really clear the streets of a lot of stupid people if I was able to do that.

Picture the scene: there I am, driving through the streets of London in a big white van, with blue flashing lights, loud sirens running and the word Ambulance written in rather large letters. As a pedestrian, what . . . would you do? Would you think 'Hmm, being run over by that would really hurt, I think I'll wait the 12 nanoseconds that it takes him to drive past before I cross the road'. Or would you, as most of the people in my area apparently do, think 'Hmm, an ambulance on his way to an important job, I bet I can run across the road in front of him before he can hit me'.

During the last job, three people tried to dive under my ambulance. If I was allowed (by government grant or some such) to keep driving and splat them across my windscreen, that would mean three less idiots being allowed to breed tonight.

Oh well, I might get lucky later tonight.

🚑 DEAR MR ALCOHOLIC

. . . Can all alcoholics please just get drunk in their houses and fall asleep there? Why do you insist that you drink your Tennent's Super in a public place where some do-gooder will think you are ill and call for an ambulance?

. . . Can you also have a bath once in a while? I know it's nice to roll around in the road while drunk, but it would be nice if you were at least a bit clean to start with.

. . . Would you mind awfully not swearing at me, taking a swing at me or exposing yourself to me? I have quite enough abuse from the non-drunks out there . . . Still at least your fists are easy to dodge, and if I stop holding you up, you fall over.

. . . If you have a medical condition, please don't use it as an excuse to get taken into hospital. If you tell me 'I'm drunk and need to sleep it off', I have less work to do than if you tell me that you have 'Chest pain, Angina, Cancer and Difficulty in Breathing'. The more tests I have to do the longer it will be before you get to hospital, and the more I have to come into physical contact with you. If you are just drunk, then I can just be a taxi.

. . . When you have been sick, at some point in the next week or so could you please change your clothing? Give them to someone who hasn't knackered their brain on booze to wash. Dry vomit on the clothing, while advertising your love for beer, doesn't endear you to me thankyouverymuch.

. . . Please keep your weight down either through diet or through terminal liver failure. I'm the poor bastard that has to lug the dead weight of your unconscious body into the ambulance.

. . . You don't have to tell me 'I'm an alcoholic', and sound so proud about it. I *do* have a nose, and can smell for myself.

. . . Finally, although Tennent's Super Strong lager, White Lightning, and for the rare rich alcoholic Stella Artois are perfectly acceptable drinks, could you please come up with something less damaging? I think lighter fuel is better for you and contains fewer chemicals.

🚐 A CHILD IS BORN . . .

The story of the first baby I delivered—I can still remember it now. I can also remember my feeling of relief when it all went smoothly. Yet still managed to turn it into a rant about midwifery.

Just in from my late-shift and feeling more upbeat than normal. Tonight I delivered my first baby . . . and yet I can still turn this happy event into a rant.

Picture the scene: you are a midwife (this means you have a chip on your shoulder the size of the African debt), and a lady comes in to your maternity department in the second stage of labour. Do you . . .

(a) Say hello, take a room and we'll have that baby out as soon as we can,

or . . .

(b) Tell them to go home and come back when the pain gets worse.

Guess which answer results in your baby being delivered by an ambulance bloke who has 1 day's training in maternity (and who, to be honest, slept through most of it)?

Then when I take mother and baby into the same maternity department are you . . .

(a) Vaguely apologetic, or . . .

(b) Snotty towards the ambulance crew who did your work for you?

Can you guess that tonight I got (b) for both questions?

Otherwise it was a nice simple delivery, with dad shooting pictures on his mobile phone sending them to all and sundry while his wife was lying, bloodstained and naked on a leather sofa. Blood went all over that sofa, which come summer will start to smell just a little rank. Blood also went all over me (note to self—must remember to pack Wellington boots next time) and my acting skills ('Don't worry mum, all normal, I've done hundreds of deliveries') were tested to the limit.

. . . and I didn't have to pick up any alcoholics.

WHY WOULD PEOPLE EVEN THINK IT?

I have sometimes been astounded by the bloodymindedness of people, and sometimes by their stupidity. Now I am astonished at their petty nastiness.

I'm driving my 'big-white-van-with-blue-flashing-lights-and-a-siren' to a 1-year-old child with difficulty in breathing. While passing a group of youths on the pavement, one of them thinks that it would be a good idea to throw his bottle of coke at the ambulance, thus spraying my screen, obscuring my vision and nearly causing me to swerve into oncoming traffic.

All I can say is that it is lucky for them that I was going to a call, because if I hadn't I'd have shoved my boot up their arse.

Where in the tiny recesses of their minds does it seem like a good idea to throw something at an ambulance running on lights and sirens?

All I hope is that one day they need me—something likely, given the amount of people like that who get stabbed in my neck of the woods—and I'm just that little too slow to save their worthless skins.

🚑 PAYMENT POINT

I get called to a lot of RTAs (that is, for the uninformed, 'Road Traffic Accident'). I'd say that 90% of these are diagnosed as 'whiplash' (which is a muscular sprain of the neck—this is a minor injury that is treated with painkillers); I'd suggest that over half of these are an attempt to gain insurance money. In the ambulance trade we call this the 'Payment Point', referring to the point in the neck that is painful, and pays out the money.

Tonight I saw the most blatant attempt to get money from an 'accident'.

I was called to a flyover where two cars had been in a near collision, yes, a near collision. There was no damage to either vehicle, neither were there any skidmarks on the road. The 'patient' was the passenger of the car, and complained of pain on the right side of his neck. He was desperate to go to hospital, for what reason I did not know, as there was obviously no injury.

This was made even more evident when he forgot what side of his neck the pain was on. When I called him on this he pretended not to know what I was talking about.

Even the police were not above making fun of this idiot.

It probably didn't help that he was 10 years younger than me and cruising around in a red sports car.

Of course RTA is now RTC (Road Traffic Collision), because if it's an 'accident' then the police can't prosecute anyone.

☕ SINGLE

Although I do love my job dearly, there are a number of disadvantages. At the moment I am a 'relief' worker, which means although I have a main station, I can be sent anywhere in London to cover absences and holidays in the 'core' staff. I also don't have a regular crewmate . . . I am essentially the whore of the London Ambulance Service.

So, at the moment I am sitting on my backside at my main station with no-one to work with, watching daytime TV.

☕ BORED, BORED, BORED, BORED . . .

Of course, at some point in the next 12 hours I could be rushing off anywhere in London. Being on strange stations is actually quite good fun, as you get to meet new people and, let's face it, in this job moving around London just means 'same shit, different scenery'.

. . . But at the moment I'm bored . . .

Daytime TV, the ambulance relief's worst enemy. Thankfully I'm no longer a relief—I'm 'Core' staff now, which means I have a regular partner and I work mainly out of one station.

10

🚐 SOME PEOPLE JUST CAN'T WAIT

So, there I am in my ambulance helping a bloke who was actually quite ill, when all of a sudden the back doors fly open and some idiot decides to start berating me because I'm blocking the road. Needless to say I am not pleased at this, not only because it is embarrassing for the patient, but also because of the sheer bloody cheek of this person. When I tell her (very politely mind you) to bugger off, she replies with the old favourite 'I'm a taxpayer and I pay your wages'. At this I remind her that my patient, my crewmate and I also pay taxes. At this she is a bit nonplussed, yet still she continues to moan that there is no need for me to block the road.

In any event, I did need to block the road, I don't do it on purpose, but it is more important to get to the patient quickly.

This woman's moaning then gets other drivers upset and they start honking their horns, and the only way I get rid of the woman who was in such a hurry was to pull the door shut after me and tell her to imagine her relative in the ambulance . . .

I didn't hurry treating the patient either.

The same thing has happened on more than one occasion. Now I simply ask the complainer that if it was them rolling around in agony, would they like to have to wait while I find a better place to park?

🚐 MAYBE IT'S BECAUSE I'M A LONDONER

Research carried out by the London Ambulance Service for our 'No Send' policy has shown that 59% of Londoners think that they will get seen

11

quicker in A&E (Accident and Emergency department) if they arrive in an ambulance.

This . . . Is . . . Not . . . True . . .

In fact, if you come to A&E after calling an ambulance for something minor, the nursing staff will be more inclined to send you out to the waiting room and forget about you.

I was an A&E nurse for a long time—just trust me on this . . .

Also, Londoners call for three times the number of ambulances for 'flu than in any other English city. Half the time the patient has got a cold and not 'flu at all, and just needs to work it out of their system. Even if they did have 'flu, there is little the hospital could do for them anyway.

Coupled with high population densities, lack of staff and vehicles, speed bumps everywhere and heavy traffic, is it any wonder we are having trouble hitting the 8-minute deadline we have to make 75% of calls in?

NICE NEW MOTORS

The London Ambulance Service is giving us poor ambulance staff shiny new ambos to drive . . . well, puke yellow rather than shiny . . . but they *are* new. These are Mercedes Sprinters outfitted in 'EURO RAL 1016 Yellow' which is apparently the most striking colour available and is used throughout the European Union. They have lots of nice new bits for us to play with. Most importantly, they have a tail lift so now we don't need to break our backs lifting some 20-stone lump into the back of the motor (20 stone is 127 kilograms for those using 'new money').

I was asked by a friend what I thought of them, and having just finished my 'Familiarisation Course' (4 hours of playing with the new toy) I must say I do like it. Not only is the engine more responsive when moving off, but the brakes also work that bit better than our old LDVs (Leyland Daf vans) and the interior is much more professional looking.

The only real problem I foresee is that the tail-lift needs around 4 yards to unload the trolley and around London this means that we will have to park in the middle of the road, blocking off other traffic. So, if you do see one of us blocking your way, please realise that there is no way we can park the things and be sure of being able to load a patient on board as well.

These things also cost £105 000 each and if we get the slightest scratch on them they have to be taken off the road and repaired (unlike the ones we have at the moment where they are beaten up until they stop working). Since our insurance has a £5 000 excess it'll mean a lot more money going to vehicle maintenance.

Should be fun, but I can't see management ever letting me drive one . . . I estimate if I can squeeze through gaps by driving until I hear the crunch . . .

While I thought that parking to allow the tail lifts space would be a big problem, our biggest problem would turn out to be the regular breaking down of the lifts.

☕ MY (SO-CALLED) EXCITING LIFE

I had my hair cut today, which has become a

weighty decision in my mind. It goes something like this . . .

(a) Do I get a crop or not? If I get a crop I'll look like I've just been released from a concentration camp; if I don't then I'll look like a paedophile.

(b) Will my mum like it? If not then I'll have to put up with 3 weeks' worth of moaning about how terrible I look.

(c) Will this cut enhance my ability to attract members of the opposite sex? To be honest, no haircut has ever done this but I live in hope.

(d) If I go to my local hairdressers will I get the trainee . . . and if I do will it be possible to get a refund?

Anyway, I went in and got a 'short-back-and-sides' and rather unfortunately I'm deaf as a post when I'm not wearing my glasses (for those who have 20/20 vision, you don't wear your glasses when getting a haircut). So when the whole place erupted in fits of laughter I didn't know if it was because of a rapidly growing bald-spot.

(*Still while I can't see it, it doesn't exist.*)

The best I can say is that I'm not having to brush my hair out of my eyes with a pair of gloves covered in someone else's vomit.

Which is nice . . .

BLOODY CAT . . .

I'm sitting here single on station (you need two people to man an ambulance, and if you haven't got anyone to work with you are 'single' and therefore unable to work. However, you need to stay on station in case they find someone else in

14

London who is single. In that case you find yourself trekking across London to work in a place you've only seen on telly). I'm hungry and bored, partly because it's night-time, and partly because there is no-one else on station.

However I have a plan . . .

To counter the boredom I have a DVD I can watch on the station's new DVD player (bought out of staff funds, so no we haven't been defrauding the NHS). The hunger problem will soon be solved by the microwave curry I have sitting in my car.

Let us now introduce a new member into the cast: when I said I was alone that was a bit of a lie, there is the station cat. Well at least I think it's a cat as it is so threadbare it could be anything. This cat is so stupid it lies in front of your ambulance just when you need it the most, and refuses to move until you physically have to ~~kick~~ lift it gently out of the way. However, it is intelligent enough to realise that when someone is using the microwave there will be an opportunity to beg for food 5 minutes later (13 minutes if the food is frozen).

I nearly fell over the damn thing stepping away from the microwave, only to spend the next 10 minutes discussing with a mouth full of chicken korma why it wouldn't like to jump up on my lap and make off with my dinner. It went a little something like this . . .

Miaow.

'No you can't have any.'

Miaow.

'You wouldn't like it.'

Miaow.

'Go eat your own dinner.'

Miaow.

Gets up, plate in hand, to check that the cat does indeed have food/water/toy mouse.

Miaow.

'Will you bugger off!'

Miaow.

At this point I put the plate (still with some of my food on it) on the floor, which the mangy beast sniffs and turns his nose up at. Said 'cat' then goes and hides under a table.

Horrible bloody creature.

It's now dead; there is only one person on station who misses the bloody thing.

WHY THIS IS A GOOD JOB

My crewmate and I went to a man having a fit on Christmas day; he was a security guard and built like a brick out-house. This fit wasn't your 'normal' epileptic fit, but instead the man was punchy and aggressive. To say it was a struggle to get him on the back of the ambulance is to say that Paris Hilton may have appeared in an Internet video download. Cutting a long story short, the patient is diabetic and his blood sugar has dropped to a dangerously low level. Luckily, we carry an injection to reverse this, and after wrestling with him in order to give him this drug he made a full recovery before we even reached the hospital. This is a nice job because we actually helped someone rather than just drove them to hospital.

Other benefits of the job include (but are not limited to . . .)

Working outside in the fresh air, I don't know

how office workers put up with air conditioning.

For much of the time you are your own boss—do not underestimate this.

Driving on the wrong side of the road with blue lights and sirens going; it's not about the speed, it's about the *power*.

Being able to poke around people's houses and feel superior even though you haven't done the washing up in your own house for 2 days.

No matter how annoying the patient is, knowing that within 20 minutes it'll be the hospital's problem.

Meeting lots of lovely nurses, and knowing that I get paid more than them.

On the rare occasion, being able to help people who are scared or in pain.

Every time I have a bad day, or feel fed up at work I think back to this list and soon start to feel better— although I no longer get paid more than the nurses I meet.

DEATH AND WHAT FOLLOWS

There are some people, who despite being lovely people, you dread working with; one such person is Nobby (not his real name). He is what is known in the trade as a 'trauma magnet'. He's one of those people who will get the cardiac arrests, car crashes, shootings and stabbings; by contrast I am a 'shit magnet', meaning I only seem to pick up people who don't need an ambulance. Other than having to do some real work for a change I really enjoy working with him.

I was working with him a little time ago and we

got called to a suspended (basically this is someone whose heart isn't beating and they have stopped breathing). It's one of those jobs that require us to work hard trying to save the punter's life. We got to the address and found relatives performing CPR on their granny. You might have seen it on TV as a 'Cardiac Arrest'.

(*Let me correct a few ideas you might have about resuscitation. First, it rarely works; 'Casualty' and 'ER' have led people to believe that you often save people: I can count on the fingers of one hand the number of people who have survived an arrest and most of them arrested while I was watching them in hospital. Second, it isn't pretty: when someone arrests there is often vomit, faeces, urine and blood covering them and the area around them. Finally, people never suspend where you can reach them: if there is an awkward hole, or they can find some way to collapse under a wardrobe they will do so.*)

This poor woman was covered in body fluids and was properly dead; there was no way we were going to save her. One of our protocols says that we can recognise someone as beyond hope and not even commence a resuscitation attempt. Unfortunately, we couldn't do it this time as the relatives had been doing CPR (which is the right thing to do) and so we had to make an attempt.

Nobby and I got to work and tried to resuscitate the patient for 30 minutes. Our protocol goes on to say that if we are unsuccessful after attempting a resuscitation for 'a specified time' we can end it and recognise death, which is what we did.

However, during our resuscitation attempt it seemed that the entire extended family had arrived and there were well over 20 people in this little

18

terraced house with much wailing and gnashing of teeth. It's always hard to tell someone that their mother had died, but it has to be done, and if you can manage it well you can answer some of their questions and hopefully provide some healing for them.

The GP (general practitioner) was informed, as were the police (a formality in sudden deaths). The family had called a priest and he was there before the police arrived, while the GP was going to 'phone the family'; what he expected to be able to do over the phone puzzled me.

We tided up and went on to another job.

Two weeks later, Nobby was called to a chest pain. He turns up and finds himself in the middle of a wake, surrounded by twenty familiar-looking people.

Can you guess who the wake was for? Its a funny old world . . .

I worked with Nobby again for the first time in 2 years. He still remembered the job, and what happened after it. I told Nobby that he'd be included in this book but he wasn't happy with his pseudonym and told me that he would prefer to be referred to as 'George Clooney'. I refused.

I DO LIKE SOME DRIVERS . . .

Although I often moan about the idiocy of other people's driving when faced with a big white van with blue flashing lights on top, I am sometimes pleasantly surprised at the lengths some people will go to in order to get out of the way. For example, yesterday we had people nearly grounding their cars on roundabouts and roadside verges, squeezing into parking spots I wouldn't be able to fit a Mini Cooper in and swearing at other drivers who wouldn't move out of the way. I've had workmen stand in the middle of the road and stop traffic, lollipop ladies fence off crossings with their 'lollipops', and van drivers who I have clipped while squeezing past them wave me on and tell me, 'don't worry about a little damage'.

Yesterday we had all the above on one call (except hitting a van driver), it was like the Red Sea parting before us. It was a beautiful thing to behold; it left us in awe and wonder.

Shame we were going to 2-year-old with a cough. *This is a rare occurrence.*

🚐 THE DANGERS OF PROSTITUTION

Occasionally you get a job that makes you laugh, normally because the person you are picking up is an idiot. We got called to a chip shop in one of the main roads in Newham—unfortunately there are about 20 chip shops on this road, but we managed to narrow it down by looking for the shiny white police car parked outside. The call had been given as an 'assault' which can mean anything from a slap on the face to a fatal stabbing.

In this instance it was a young lad, the spitting image of 'Ali G', who was complaining that he had been hit on the nose; needless to say there wasn't a mark on him, and it turned out that he had been hit by his girlfriend. The police wanted to take statements, but he wasn't interested and when I tried to assess him he told me that the ambulance wasn't needed as 'I'm St Johns innit, and a security guard'. This fella couldn't scare a toddler, so I suspected he was telling a little bit of a lie. As he wasn't hurt and 'refused aid' my crew-mate and I retreated to a safe distance to do our paperwork . . .

In the course of the night we found ourselves at the local hospital (dropping off yet another ill person) when who should walk in with another crew from my station, but our earlier 'Ali G' lookalike. I asked him why he decided to call an ambulance when he'd already sent us packing and it turned out that another woman had hit him . . . the prostitute he'd hired after his girlfriend had slapped him. Turns out she had hit him and then robbed him of his jewellery. He couldn't have put up much of a fight because he only had one scratch on him.

It's pillocks like these we have to put up with . . . and call 'sir' . . .

However, it is also jobs like this that we can use to have a good laugh with our workmates. So people like him do serve some purpose.

🚑 MY NIGHT SHIFT

Much fun and games last night, working in the Poplar/Bow area. Not only did some German bloke graffiti on the back of one of the ambulances, but he also called the crew from a payphone and ran off, repeating it twice.

There are a *lot* of strange people out there . . .

MacMedic (an American ambulance blog) gave a rundown of what his shifts are like, so I thought

21

I'd do the same, in honour of our brothers in foreign climes.

All these people called an ambulance last night by dialling '999'.

(a) Fractured wrist—young lad at the Boat Show.

(b) An alcoholic 'frequent flyer' who has just been released from prison . . . We thought we'd got rid of him for good.

(c) A 15-year-old with a runny nose.

(d) Very minor RTA.

(e) Domestic Assault, with no actual injury, but police already on scene.

(f) 'Facial Injury' which turned out to mean 'Some bloke kicked my door'.

(g) Assault with a cut hand—actually a decent injury with tendon involvement (which means surgery and physiotherapy).

(h) Varicose Vein that had burst—plenty of blood everywhere.

(i) A 29-year-old with chest pain, hyperventilating, with very upset relatives.

(j) A suicidal overdose in a house filled with young men with short hair and tight T-shirts (ifyouknowwhatImean).

(k) RTA with a traffic light pole coming off the worse in a two-car collision.

(l) An 8-month pregnant female who had fallen earlier that day.

and . . .

(m) A fitting 9-year-old; only one parent spoke English, and they decided to stay at home and send the father who *doesn't* speak English with us, because 'The hospital has interpreters . . .'

Now, out of these thirteen jobs, only five actually

went to hospital . . .

This counts as a 'good shift', reasonably interesting jobs, and no-one tried to hit me.

🚑 I HATE PSYCHIATRIC 'SERVICES'

Sorry folks, bit of a rant here . . . but I last slept 22 hours ago . . .

We got a call to a patient who was 'Depressed—not moving': normally with this type of call it's some teenager having a strop, but this time it was a little different. Basically, the patient, who suffers from depression, was discharged from the local psychiatric unit 3 weeks ago and recently had her dose of antidepressants reduced. Yesterday, she was crying all night, and tonight she was just sitting staring into space, refusing to make eye contact and not talking at all.

One of the things that we as an ambulance crew cannot do is physically remove someone to hospital if they don't want to go—that would be kidnapping and is frowned upon by the law. This young girl was not going anywhere despite my best attempts to persuade her—she just wasn't communicating.

The solution would be simple: call the Community Psychiatric Nursing (CPN) team to come and assess her and, if needed, arrange her compulsory removal to the psychiatric unit (called a 'Section' under the Mental Health Act). The problem? It was 10 p.m. . . .

First off I phoned the psychiatric unit that she had received treatment under. After talking to two idiots who had trouble understanding plain English, I finally managed to get the number of the

23

CPN team. Now, the London Ambulance Service (LAS) is quite smart: when we want to arrange an outside agency we go through our Control because all the telephone conversations are recorded . . . so if someone says they are going to attend they damn well better. I got onto Control, passed the details to them and waited for them to get back to us.

I'd just like to say that in all my years of medical experience I have never had a simple referral to a psychiatric service: they always seem to try shirking any form of work by 'forgetting' you or by being just plain obstructive. Maybe I'm just lucky and get the idiots every time.

Needless to say we waited . . . and waited . . . and waited . . . from 22:20 until 23:00 we waited; then at 23:02 Control got back to us. Apparently the CPN team all goes home at 23:00 and hadn't answered the phone until 23:00 on the dot. So they refused to visit the patient. The moral so far is if you are going to have a psychiatric breakdown in Newham don't do it after 22:00.

So we switched to plan 'B', which is to arrange the out-of-hours social worker to come and visit, as they double as Psychiatric Liaison. Again we went through Control and waited . . . and waited . . . and waited . . . Finally we heard back that the social worker would ring the family and would like to talk to me. (Outside agencies try this trick, as they know the patient's phone isn't being recorded, and so can say whatever they want, with any disagreement being my word against theirs.) The social worker explained that she was very busy and so would prefer not to come to see the patient and have I tried the out-of-hours GP?

Back to Control I went and got them to try and

24

contact the out-of-hours GP (a GP, for those not in the UK, is the patient's family doctor). Can you guess what we then did? We waited . . . and waited . . . and waited . . . Finally, Control got back to us and informed us that the out-of-hours GP hadn't arrived for work yet and that when they did, they would have to see two other patients first.

All through this time the family of the patient were very understanding and were happy when I explained that the GP would call at some point in the night. All I could do was advise them to remove anything that the patient could use to hurt herself, and keep an eye on her, calling us back if they felt the need.

Total amount of time an ambulance was tied up trying to get outside agencies to DO THEIR DAMN JOB—2 hours and 19 minutes . . . and not the world's most satisfactory outcome.

As I mentioned to our Control, sometimes you feel very lonely out there on the mean streets of Newham.

It is still the case that as soon as the sun goes down, various community services disappear and people in trouble need to rely on the ambulance service and the A&E department, even if it isn't the best place for them.

STICKY FEET

There is something deeply disturbing about walking on a sticky carpet—especially when the flat is in a complete mess and the punter has called an ambulance four times in the last 2 days for a pain in the chest that has lasted *2 years*. I'd like the jury to note that the pain hasn't changed in any way, it's not worse, or moved around the body, he has no other symptoms. But the patient just seems to like calling ambulances. I wanted to wipe my feet on the way out of the flat.

It also doesn't help when the patient smells so bad that I want to leap out the side window. We didn't have any air freshener (and apparently, neither does the hospital).

When we got to the hospital the triage nurse took one look at the patient, muttered 'Not him again' and sent him out to the waiting room. I suspect that it may just be a ploy to use biological warfare to empty the waiting room.

I still keep getting called back to him for the exact same 'problem'.

🚑 WORKLOAD

Once again I know a lot of visitors here are from America, so I'm going to explain how the LAS works on a day-to-day basis. This will either be very boring or immensely interesting—your choice.

Ambulances run out of dedicated stations, we don't share stations with the Fire Service. In fact, some years ago, when it was suggested the idea was shot down as we would be disturbing the firecrews' sleep throughout the night. Each station has its own call-sign 'K1', 'J2', 'G4' for example, then each ambo has a suffix that is attached to this, so one ambulance running out of station J2 would be called J201, while another would be J207.

The stations are spaced approximately 5–6 miles apart, and you mainly service the area surrounding the station; however, with interhospital transfers and other irregularities you can quite easily find yourself across the other side of London.

It's an old joke that when asking if we need to travel so far the dispatcher will ask us if it still says London *on the side of the ambulance.*

There is a main station, and two or three 'satellite' stations; the main station will normally have between three and six ambulances running from it, while the smaller stations have between one and four. There is less cover at night, and you can easily find yourself being the only ambulance running from a given station.

Across London we deal with more than 3 500 calls per day, and with a fleet of 400 ambulances of which perhaps only three-quarters are manned, we seldom get a rest. Where I work we average one job an hour, and are supposed to transport every one of those patients to hospital.

The longest shift we officially do is 12 hours, in which we can expect 10–13 jobs, which doesn't sound like a lot but is enough to keep us busy . . . We spend 97% of our time away from station (compared with 3% for the fire service).

However, it *is* a fun job.

☕ NIGHT SHIFTS

There has been a discussion over on another medical blog's forums over which shift we prefer to work. Like many of the others I have a preference for working though the night. The reasons for this are many but include:

(1) I'm single, I can lie in bed as long as I want.

And breakfast is dinner . . . and kebabs are lunch . . . and an icecream is supper.

(2) You get empty streets, and so can drive like someone out of 'The Fast and the Furious'.

(3) You also get the strange jobs: 'sex-toy accidents', criminal behaviour, stabbings . . .

(4) It feels as if you 'own' the world: there is no-one else around, and anyone you do meet is normally shocked to be awake at night.

(5) You get to work a lot of jobs with the police, who are generally excellent people to work with.

(6) I get to sleep through early morning television—I'm sorry but I can't see the attraction of 'Trisha' or 'This Morning'.

(7) I don't have to go into a school, and be surrounded by 400 screaming children just because a kid has sprained their ankle.

(8) There is less management around—actually there is no management around (always a good thing); I like to avoid management as much as I can: I worked this job for 6 months before they remembered my name.

(9) On a cold winter morning, I'm going home to my warm comfortable bed, while everyone else is trudging to work.

I still like nights, which makes me a rarity in the LAS. Most of my most interesting jobs occur at night.

BUSY, BUSY, BUSY

No sooner do I post why I like nightshifts than I get two 'proper' emergency calls, one after another. The first was a 76-year-old Male 'Suspended'. Unfortunately, despite our best efforts there was little hope for him, and he died later in hospital without his heart ever restarting. His wife of 50 or more years was disbelieving of the whole situation, and I was too busy doing CPR to be able to comfort her much. It is one of the few things that I miss about nursing—sometimes you want to spend time with a relative. If you can't do anything for the patient, the relatives then become your concern. For the first time in 50 years she was going to sleep alone and the nurse who would be looking after her is not someone that I would call the most sympathetic person in the world. I spent a little longer at hospital talking to the wife. The only consolation that I could give her was something that I've practised many times over the years—that her husband never suffered, and that he wouldn't have felt anything that we did. Large amount of blood over the tarmac. He could have been worse—he was lying in the middle of the road and could have easily been run over. It is important in such a job that you should 'collar and board' them. This is a way of immobilising someone in order to prevent any damage to the spinal cord. Unfortunately the patient was quite combative and so the only safe way to secure his head was for me to hold it during the transport—all the time blood was leaking through the dressing we had put on him, all over us, the trolley bed and the floor of the ambulance. Some managed to flick up onto my crewmate's face, which is something you don't really want happening to you.

I've just come back from the hospital (after dropping off yet another assault) and our patient is doing fine—seems that his altered consciousness was indeed as a result of the alcohol. He still isn't sober enough to have a meaningful conversation, but he is looking a lot better than when we picked him up.

I still like wrestling with drunks, and writing about blood being flicked up into your face set the stage for a future set of posts.

NEW UNIFORMS (BUT STILL GREEN)

The LAS has got some new uniforms. These include 'combat trousers' and a fleece, which is nice seeing as it can get a bit nippy around here. The only problem is that we use 'Alexandra', who doesn't have the best reputation for our uniforms. We'll forget that they can't measure you up correctly—I am not a 38-inch waist no matter how many kebabs I eat. Instead, let us consider that the buttons on their shirts tend to fall off at the worse possible moment. Having a button drop in a dead man's mouth when you are trying to resuscitate him is not something that inspires confidence in the relatives watching. I was supposed to have eight shirts; two of them have been cannibalised, so that I have six shirts with the right number of buttons.

The new uniform actually seems quite nice. We have a little NHS logo in case the big motor with 'Ambulance' written on the side is not enough of a clue to our identity, and the shirts have a mesh in the armpits so we can let our sweat out. The combat trousers have 'Permagard' (their spelling, not mine) which is designed to kill bacteria, which is nice considering the state of some of the houses we visit. The high-visibility jackets are . . . well . . . visible and we now have a green 'beanie hat' (I

30

think it's green so that people won't wear them anywhere except at work).

There is a rumour that we will be getting new boots soon . . . 'Magnums'. We are a bit like the army in that we buy our own boots because the ones supplied are a bit shoddy.

Anyway the uniform 'goes live' on the 12th but those who have uniform that actually fits have been wearing them early. The bosses are moaning a bit but haven't actually told anyone off about it.

I now have five shirts with the right number of buttons. People are still buying their own boots.

DADDY, DAUGHTER, KILL

Picked up an assault yesterday. While sitting in the back of the ambulance he told his 2-year-old daughter that 'daddy is gonna fucking kill the people who did this to me', then complained when the nurse at the hospital told him to moderate his language.

I love this job.

We then went to someone who started hitting his own nose in order to prove that it had been bleeding earlier, and then went to a woman who had a bleeding varicose vein that had stopped bleeding, but wanted to pick at it to prove that it had been bleeding.

Then went to a 14-year-old girl who was 'fitting' but when we got there was confused and combative—she was a diabetic so we checked her blood sugar, which was low. Being confused is one of the symptoms of a low blood sugar and we normally give them an injection that brings them out of it. We gave the injection and waited for it to work and receive the grateful thanks of the parents.

But it didn't work.

We checked the blood sugar again, and it had come back up to normal levels, yet the condition of the girl was unchanged.

So we (rather quickly) took her into hospital— we haven't been back there yet to find out what had caused her confusion. Was it drugs, alcohol, psychiatric problems, CVA (cerebrovascular accident) or even just a bad nightmare? Once we get back to the hospital which we took her to we will no doubt be able to find out. She didn't have a high temperature, didn't have any medical history besides the diabetes, her pupils were normal and responsive; all observations were normal.

We spend a lot of time dealing with things that are simple to cope with. You can fix them almost by rote thinking, but every so often you get a job that throws you off balance. Normally you 'wake up' and deal with it by going back to basics, but other jobs just completely confuse you, and this was one of those jobs.

This post got me a large number of people coming to my site looking for the search term 'Daddy fucking daughter'. Sometimes the Internet is a scary place. It turned out that the girl had been drinking vodka, and that this was the reason behind her confused and combative state

☕ ORCON!

ORCON—the biggest problem with the ambulance service, and the biggest cause of staff/management friction. Every so often I will revisit this topic, as it's of such importance.

I'm single at work at the moment (which means I don't have anyone to work with—so am sitting on station twiddling my thumbs), so I thought I'd tell you all about the great God ORCON and how he rules the life of every EMT/paramedic in England.

This is really boring, so I'll not be hurt if you don't bother reading any further.

The government likes to give everything targets, from school grades, the waiting time for breast cancer referrals to the number of trains on time.

The ambulance service has only one main target to reach, that of ORCON. ORCON was started in 1974 and governs how fast we are expected to respond to 'Cat A' calls. ('Cat A' calls are our high-priority calls, although because of the way calls are assessed, they are rarely seriously ill patients).

Essentially, for every 'Cat A' call in London we have to be there within 8 minutes.

Simple really.

It doesn't matter what actually happens to the patient, just so long as we get there within 8 minutes. For example, if we get to someone who has been dead for 2 days within 8 minutes, that counts as a *Success*. If we get to a heart attack in 9 minutes, provide life-saving treatment and ensure that their quality of life is a good as possible it counts as a *Failure*.

For those who don't live in London, let's just say that traffic is often heavy, and there are speed-bumps and tiny side-roads. We have more than 300 languages spoken in London, which may delay getting the location we are needed at. We are hideously overused and understaffed, we face delays at hospital owing to overcrowding and delays on-scene because of the ignorant people we have to attend to.

None of this matters—all that matters is the 8-minute deadline. If we make 75% of all calls in 8 minutes we get more money from the government, which means more staff, vehicles that work etc. . . . If we don't make 75% then we don't get any more money and we continue to struggle. This year it looks like we are going to make it, but only just.

There isn't any reason behind 8 minutes being the time we need to get to people: brain death occurs after 4 minutes or so; trauma, while needing to be treated as quickly as possible, has the 'Golden Hour'. The current rumour is that it is how long MPs have to vote when the Division Bell rings in parliament—who knows? No-one I have spoken to has any decent answers.

Well, that should be the last of my posts on the boring 'day to day' running of the London Ambulance Service.

You may all rejoice now.

🚑 OH . . . BOLLOCKS . . .

Rather obviously this topic dominated my weblog for some time—I'm including only some of it here, because I'm sure that you didn't want to pay good money to read about me being horribly ill. I haven't edited this post for this book—it's much how it originally appeared on my website. I started writing it less than 2 hours after I was exposed.

There is a fear that every health-care worker has. Tonight that fear jumped up and slapped me in the face.

Second job of the shift, we were called to '50-year-old male—collapsed in street'. Normally this is someone who is drunk, but we rushed to the scene anyway, just in case it isn't (we rush to *everything*—it's the only way to be sure you are not caught out). We reach the scene and see the male laying on the floor talking gibberish. He is bleeding from a cut on his face and possibly from his jaw. Bystanders tell us that he 'just dropped'. He then starts to vomit, and because it's dark we get him on our trolley and into the back of the ambulance.

Our basic assessment finds that he has no muscular tone on his right side, although all his observations are within normal limits. Deciding against hanging around we start transport to hospital. Halfway to hospital he starts to vomit and cough—part of this vomitus/blood flies unerringly across the width of the ambulance . . .

. . . right into my open mouth.

Pretty disgusting, but what can you do? The patient then starts to come around, now able to move all limbs and to talk. This is good, it means I'm able to get some history from him. So I get his name, date of birth, address. Then I ask this 50-year-old if he is normally fit and well.

'No', he says, 'I have AIDS (acquired immune-deficiency syndrome)'.

Bollocks.

I've never had anything from a patient in my mouth before (apart from the odd chocolate when I was a nurse), so of course the first time is with an HIV (human immunodeficiency virus)-positive patient.

My crewmate looks in the rear view mirror, and that look passes between us. Ambulance people will know what I mean—it's the 'Oh shit' look that you give/get when something goes horribly wrong.

We get to the hospital and the patient is looking a lot better, fully orientated, full strength and starting to feel the pain from a probably busted jaw. So I get to hand over to the nurse, which turned into a bit of a comedy moment . . .

Me: 'Patient witnessed collapse, had right-sided hemiparesis, now resolved. Previous history includes AIDS'.

Handover Nurse: 'Fine'

Charge Nurse: 'You can't say that'

Me: 'Pardon?'

Charge Nurse: 'You can't say AIDS—people will be prejudiced against him'

Me: 'Well they shouldn't be, and this is medical stuff. It's a syndrome like any other'

Charge Nurse: 'You have to call it something else'

Me: 'I don't really care for political correctness, besides I'm a patient as well—I swallowed some of his blood'

Charge Nurse: 'Oh, well . . . lets get you sorted out then'

I then went through the rigmarole of having blood taken, then I asked to be put on PEP, which the charge nurse agreed I should be put on. PEP is 'Post Exposure Prophylaxis'—basically a cocktail of antiretroviral drugs that, taken over a 4-week period, will hopefully reduce any live virus to non-infective amounts. Common side-effects include nausea, vomiting, headache, diarrhoea, cough, abdominal pain/cramps, muscle pain, tiredness, flu-like symptoms, difficulty in sleeping, rash and (*I love this one*) flatulence.

Other more uncommon side-effects are . . . pancreatitis, anaemia, neutropenia, peripheral neuropathy, and other 'metabolic effects'.

I'm in for a barrel of laughs for these next 4 weeks . . .

The charge nurse looked really sympathetic when he offered me stuff to look after the side-effects—he used to work in an HIV clinic so I guess he knows better than me what I'm in for . . .

Then we talked about rates of infection, which is why I'm feeling kinda relaxed here. HIV is a tough virus to catch (compared with hepatitis, which is the one that worries me). If I were to stab myself with a needle after drawing HIV-positive blood I would have a 0.004% chance of catching the virus. Swallowing a bit of blood/vomitus is less risky than that, especially as I have no mouth/stomach ulcers. With the PEP my chances of 'seroconverting' are as close to zero as you can get. I knew all this before I set foot in the hospital, which probably explained why I wasn't a quivering wreck.

So far 'only' two medical workers have seroconverted after needle-stick injuries. I greatly doubt that I'll be the third.

So 'The Plan' is that I go to see Occupational Health on Monday, and they will advise me on what happens next. I've been told already that I'll have to avoid sexual contact for the next 3 months (not a hardship—I've managed 'no sexual contact' for 2 years before now) and that I'll probably need to take 4 weeks off work due to me feeling too ill from the side-effects of the antiretrovirals.

We'll see about that . . . I don't 'do' ill.

Anyway, if I do need to take time off it'll give me a chance to read some books I've got sitting on my

shelf—and complete 'Zelda—Windwaker'.
Gotta go now, I feel flatulent already . . .
I never got around to completing 'Zelda'.

🚑 'DONOR' TAKES ON NEW MEANING

I got a lot of support over the previous post, and to be honest I would have been a lot less calm if I didn't have my blog where I could offload some of my worries.

First, thanks to everyone who has contacted me over my 'exposure', I appreciate it all, even if I haven't personally replied to you (you'll find out why I might not have answered you a bit later in this post . . .).

I went to Occupational Health on Monday, basically to let them know about my exposure, and that I was on PEP. The LAS showed how nice they are by lending me a spare ambulance to drive to my appointment—GPS navigation comes in handy when you don't know where you are going.

Occupational Health is south of the river at King's College Hospital, which is a bit of a trek. 'Occy Health' took baseline blood samples, so they would know if there was any effect on my liver/kidneys/white cell count, and filled in a couple of forms about my exposure. Then they told me that they would get in contact with the 'donor' to see what his virus load and hepatitis status was.

Until now I always thought of 'donor' as a 'nice' word—heart donors and the like—I never really thought it would happen to include this circumstance.

During the consultation they told me that I'd

need blood tests every fortnight for the next month and a half, and that my first HIV/hepatitis status check would be in 3 months, with an additional one in 6 months. Should they both be negative then I would be in the clear.

They also told me of the side-effects of the antiretrovirals that I am taking, and seemed surprised that all I was experiencing was similar to a mild hangover.

That was yesterday—today was spent vomiting/sleeping to avoid nausea/and experiencing the joys of explosive diarrhoea.

My station officer called up and asked me how I was. When I told him, he basically told me to take it easy and go back to work when I felt better.

However, there was some good news when the Occupational Health nurse contacted me, and told me that the donor's viral load was low, that there were no resistances to the PEP drugs I'm taking and that in 2002 he was free of hepatitis. That has eased my mind somewhat.

Some people have commented that I'm taking it rather well. There are a number of reasons for this, not least that the chances of me becoming HIV-positive are less than 1 in 5 000. The other thing is that I can't do anything now to change those odds, apart from continue to take the PEP.

The other side-effect of the meds I'm taking are that I'm having a certain 'vagueness': my mind isn't operating on all four cylinders, so if this seems disjointed, I've got an excuse . . .

Even today I'm not sure that the PEP drugs didn't permanently 'disjoint my mind'.

☕ PAVLOV'S DOG

Well, the PEP is still going down, unfortunately I've developed a pavlovian response to the hours of 8 o'clock. Every 12 hours I need to take the pills—I start to get nauseous just thinking about it, the familiar copper taste hits my mouth and I just want to lie down.

I also seem to have lost any control over my circadian rhythms, I'm sleeping for 14–16 hours straight and I'm drowsy for the rest—doesn't matter whether it is day or night.

At the moment the rather wonderful 'Scissor Sisters' album is chilling me out nicely, particularly 'Return to Oz' (which has a bit that puts me in mind of The Kinks' 'Lola').

I am, however, losing the motivation for cooking food, not least because of the large amount of washing up accruing in my sink. It makes me feel like a student again.

Also, my PC is screaming out for a complete overhaul—I just can't be bothered.

🚐 MOTHERING SUNDAY

Well, Saturday was the last day I worked but Greenfairy (another blogger) mentioned something that I wanted to write about—but forgot, for some bizarre reason . . .

The first call of Saturday was to a '?Suspended'. ['?Suspended' means 'Query Suspended' which means that the patient might be suspended (a.k.a 'dead')—we don't know, they might just be asleep, or drunk, or have a high temperature or a cut

40

finger, but the person calling us is a twit.]

So we hack along the road, knowing full well that because it is the first job of the day the patient is definitely going to be dead.

We arrive at the house and the FRU is there before us—I grab my kit and bound up the stairs past the daughter who called us and into the bedroom. Where a very dead lady was lying on the bed while the Rapid Responder was completing his paperwork.

One look is all you need to tell if someone has been dead for some time—and this lady had that look. It turned out that the daughter last saw her mother alive an hour ago, but that she was feeling a little unwell and took to bed. The daughter had checked on her half an hour later and found her not breathing. She then waited 20 minutes to call us as she was in such a 'tizzy'. A quick look told us that even if we had been there when it had happened it was unlikely we could do much: various clues led us to think that a stomach ulcer had ruptured and she had bled out into her stomach.

All around the house were flowers and cards—the next day being Mothering Sunday.

No sooner than we had informed the daughter that her mother had died than the doorbell went and my crewmate went down to see who it was. It was only a bleedin' flower delivery man, delivering flowers to the (now) dearly departed. My crewmate told the delivery guy that now, perhaps, wasn't the best time to bring flowers but took them in anyway, hiding them in the kitchen.

Perfect!

Then we had to wait an hour for the police to

turn up, which is normal procedure for any death in the home and is nothing to worry about. I then helped the police turn her body (to look for anything strange) and put my hand in a puddle of urine [There are two things that I can't smell— alcohol on someone's breath and urine that isn't infected with bacteria.]—something that wouldn't bother me, IF I was wearing any gloves.

Oh well.

THE OTHER GUY

I'm feeling a little better, the side-effects of the PEP seem to have subsided somewhat, although the flatulence is reaching epic proportions, which, coupled with the diarrhoea, makes every bowel motion an adventure

I have my second date with Occupational Health on Friday, for a blood test to make sure that the PEP isn't battering my liver/kidneys/pancreas and that my white cell count hasn't lowered. Work have said they'll do everything they can to supply a vehicle to get me down to south-east London.

I've been thinking a bit about the 'donor'; I wonder how he feels—he's lying in bed after having a rather frightening collapse in the street, with a broken jaw and the reason for the collapse unknown. Then a couple of days later the medical team ask him to consent to some more blood tests because he may have infected the EMT who helped him out.

If it were me I'd be absolutely mortified.

When I talk to Occupational Health I'll ask them if they can get a message back to him, letting him know that I'm fine and that I don't blame him for anything. I know his name and address, but I don't think it'd be right to turn up on his doorstep to talk to him.

I hope *he* is alright and that the collapse was something simple—I suspect a 'TIA' (transient ischaemic attack), which can be a precursor to a stroke, but with the right medications hopefully the threat of that can be controlled.

I never got to see him again, so he never found out the results of my blood tests. I kind of hope that he gets to read this, so he knows that I'm fine.

🚐 TWELVE HOURS TO GO

In 12 hours I will have stopped PEP. Those seven pills are the last ones that I am going to take.

I am extremely happy about this.

It has been a month since my stomach didn't feel as if I were waiting to vomit, a month since my thought processes have seemed even remotely like mine. A month since I last worked—good grief, am I bored! A month of wondering if my life is about to change for the worst. A month of my mates looking sideways at me when I had to take the pills in front of them (but still friends enough to laugh and joke with me about it). A month of having to get out of bed to eat breakfast, because the pills need food in my stomach. A month without shaving (why bother, I'm not allowed to have sex!). A month of feeling just the tiniest bit isolated. A month of people who I have never met, from places around the globe I have never seen, wishing me well. A month of always feeling grateful to those

43

people, for this is the kindness of strangers—in itself a random act of reality.

All over now.

In two months I get to go for my HIV test, which should be fun and giggles.

But for now—I'm happy.

I really think that if it wasn't for my blogging and the support of my friends around the globe I'd have gone mad from boredom. My next book should be 'Blogging as a Mental Health Exercise'.

🚑 PROPER DAY

My first 'proper' day back at work, working with my new crewmate on a proper ambulance.

The first job was a 66-year-old male who had been fixing tiles on his shed roof and had fallen off the ladder, probably around 10 feet. He was shut behind his front door and all I could hear through his letterbox was 'I've broken my leg'.

The police are much better than me at getting into locked premises (the last time I tried I fell on my arse in front of a crowd of 20 people) so we waited for them to arrive and use their specialised equipment (screwdriver/size 12 boot) to force open the door.

Gaining access to our customer it was pretty obvious that he had fractured his femur (thighbone) as it had a new bendy section just above the knee. The pulse was good in his foot and he didn't complain of pain anywhere else in his body. This brave man had crawled, with this fracture, from his garden through his kitchen to the living room where he kept his phone. All throughout our treatment he didn't complain once. We splinted his leg and 'collared and boarded' him from the house (a fall of 10 feet can easily break your neck, and the pain from his leg could easily distract him from a neck injury). We could have set traction on his leg, but we were only 5 minutes from the hospital; so we 'blued' him into Newham General Hospital, where he was 'attacked' by the local trauma team.

The next job we got was a dinner lady at a local primary school who had dropped a knife on her foot. There was a tiny cut to the foot, and after cleaning, dressing and checking her tetanus status we left her at work. What depressed us was that there were no scraps of food left we could have.

Driving back from the last job we saw four workmen chasing another man who ducked into the local mosque. We ignored this until we got a call to the area the men had run from—apparently a man had been assaulted with a 'Car-lock'. HEMS (our emergency helicopter service) had been activated and were going to make their way to the scene. When we did a quick U-turn and rolled up to scene it soon became obvious that HEMS was not needed so we cancelled them down. The man had been clamping an illegally parked car when the owner and his wife returned. The car owner then pulled a large aerosol can from his boot and hit our patient around the back of the neck, causing a short period of unconsciousness. His wife had also put up a fight, but the owner of the car had run (into the aforementioned mosque) leaving his wife behind. (What a gent!). At one point we thought it was going to turn into a riot as 30 youths from the mosque were adamant that the four workmen doing the chasing weren't going to set foot in the mosque.

Again, we had to collar and board him, and lift him onto our stretcher, which wasn't much fun as the man weighed at least 20 stone. Subsequent treatment at hospital showed no serious injuries.

Final job (after having to get our nice, new, shiny ambulance fixed—a problem with the side-door) was a 60-year-old female collapsed at a bus station with slurred speech and 'not drunk'. Remember that, 'not drunk', it's important.

What could it be? Could it be a stroke? Could it be hypoglycaemia? Could it be cardiac related? So we turned up to find 'Mary' having fallen over, smelling strongly of alcohol and with a 5/6ths empty bottle of whisky in her purse. (*My crewmate had to tell me about the smell of alcohol, as I've mentioned before, I'm pretty much unable to smell it myself.*)

'Not drunk'—why did the callmaker say that? It's bloody obvious she was pissed as a fart. I'd guess it was the bus station staff who wanted her gone and were afraid we wouldn't turn up if we knew she was drunk. Still, it was an easy last job of the shift, even if she did keep grabbing at my balls and kissing my (thankfully) gloved hand.

This counts as a good day.

Now I'm off for some endorphin-releasing Bailey's ice-cream.

Can you tell I was deliriously happy to be back at work?

🚑 THESE BOOTS . . .

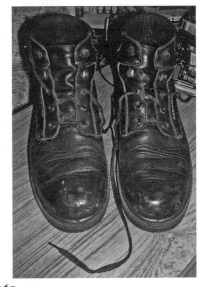

These Boots . . .
Have walked along train tracks
Have been washed in the blood of murder victims
Have kicked in doors to get to unconscious women
Have stepped in more urine, in more tower blocks, than I'd care to think about
Have kept my feet warm and comfortable on long nights
Have been allowed into a mosque
Have climbed fences to reach dead bodies
Have run across football fields to try to save a life, and failed
Have been spat on, vomited on and shat on
Have stood in 'remains'
Have tried to find purchase while walking backward down narrow stairs
Have defended me from drunks and druggies
Have been run over by a 22-stone trolley
Have been stared at by a daughter when I was telling them their mother had died
For Pixeldiva who denies she has a shoe fetish.

🚑 GAMMA GT

I went to Occupational Health today—it seems that the last time they checked my blood (because of being on PEP) my liver enzymes were a bit elevated. Most significantly my gamma-GT

47

(gamma-glutamyl transpeptidase) was at 164 (it should be between 0 and 55). PEP is well known as having effects on the liver, so this isn't completely unexpected.

More blood was taken today to check that the enzymes have returned to normal. The nurse was very concerned that I was alright in having my blood drawn, and that I wouldn't faint. She was asking me this while I'm sitting opposite her in full uniform . . .

The nurse was also a bit surprised that I'd had aural hallucinations and looked as me as if she thought I was turning schizophrenic—I assured her that the 'voices' were now leaving me alone and that it wasn't a problem. She'd never heard of this symptom before, so at least I entertained someone today.

🚐 DEAF OLD WOMEN

Nobby is working tonight from our main station. He is always a good laugh and always seems to have a joke whenever he works. Tonight I met him outside the hospital and he told me about a deaf old woman he had just brought in.

It was raining as he started to wheel her out her house so he made the comment 'It's raining, you picked a fine time to be ill'.

'Eh?' was the reply.

'The rain . . . it mucks up my hair'.

'Eh?'

'MY HAIR'

With this she took a long hard look at Nobby's very short, and very receding hair and asked him, 'Is it because of cancer?'

It is now 3:00 a.m. and already every other patient we have picked up has been drinking—from the 38-year-old male having a panic attack, who didn't want to talk to us, to the 50-year-old female who slipped on some steps coming out from the pub and cut her head. This has so far ended with our last call being one of our smelly 'frequent flyers', who thankfully decided not to hang around and wait for us to turn up.

Then there was the police car that managed to accidentally force another car into someone's garden—one of those jobs where every passing car slows down to stare. Thankfully, there were no injuries, apart from the house-owner's disturbed sleep. (At least I assume it was the owner—he was dressed in no shoes and a dressing gown).

With a bit of luck people are now wrapped up nice and snug in bed—away from the rain—and the only calls we will get will be the 5:00 a.m. 'I'm in labour' call that will result in a baby around 11:00 a.m. (long after I'm in bed).

🚐 HAND OVER MOUTH

No sooner do I hope for a quiet hour or two than the activation phone goes; it's sending us 200 yards up the road to a 'Collapsed Male'. We are met by two police officers who tell us that the patient was walking along the street, saw the policemen and then collapsed.

We get to the patient and my crewmate can't smell any alcohol on him, but he is coughing and spluttering like an Oscar winner. He complains of a headache, coughing, leg pain, back pain and an inability to walk. Other than that he is refusing to talk to us. Examination is normal and the patient is obviously play-acting.

He then does one of the things that I really hate (given the prevalence of tuberculosis in Newham); he coughs all over us and the vehicle *without putting his hand over his mouth*. Then he starts to spit on the floor of the ambulance, again something I take a dim view of—but I'm driving so I leave it to my crewmate to sort out.

Forty seconds later and we pull up outside the hospital, and our patient decides to roll around the floor. By now our patience is wearing thin, so we haul him up and throw him in a wheelchair.

In the hospital he refuses to speak to the nurses, says he cannot stand and doesn't acknowledge any requests. We leave him there and within 30 seconds are back on station.

While at the hospital I indulged in a little bit of teaching. The nurse who was assessing our patient was trying to check his pupil response (by shining a light in each eye and making sure that it reacts to light) but the eyes don't appear to be reacting. I then suggest turning off the ceiling light that the patient is lying on his back staring at.

I still have patients who insist on coughing without putting their hand over their mouth. I've given up asking them to stop—instead I just give them oxygen, via a nice tightly-fitting oxygen mask. I got a lot of people coming to this post searching for 'Hand over mouth'. I swear I don't know why.

ESSENTIAL, NOT EMERGENCY

One of the bizarre things about the Ambulance Service is that, in the eyes of the government, we are an 'essential' service but not an 'emergency' service. We are 'essential' because the emergency services (Police, Fire Brigade and Coastguard) are run by the Home Office but Ambulance Services across the country are run by NHS Trusts, and as such do not have access to the same resources as the true 'emergency' services. The distinction is often slight, but can sometimes have quite important considerations for our safety.

Last night was a case in point. We were called to a patient with abdominal pain; however, further information was given that the patient could be violent. There was something in this information that triggered my 'danger-sense', so I was happy to wait for police assistance to arrive before approaching the house.

Four police officers turned up—normally only two are sent to assist us—and they told us that their computer system, and their personal experience with the householder showed him as a nasty piece of work. We followed the police to the patient and they told him that they were going to search him, and that they wanted to put him in handcuffs first. The patient had obviously been involved with the police before, as once he was handcuffed they checked to see if he had any *new* warrants out for his arrest . . .

Searching him they found a large stick, and a rather worrying-looking (5-inch) knife on his person.

All through this the 'lady' of the house was

shouting abuse, mainly at the patient, but occasionally at the police officers present. One quick examination showed nothing life-threatening, so we offered a trip to hospital, which the patient accepted. However, as we left the house the woman shouted a few final obscenities at the patient and he then told us he couldn't be bothered to go to hospital and stalked off into the night. (*This was not a problem for either my crewmate or myself.*)

Police computers had information that he was dangerous (a number of rather vicious assaults) but our computers are not allowed to have such data. A police dispatcher has told us that they have all sorts of information on addresses, from animal liberation protesters to Members of Parliament. Again, our computers don't have any information of that sort unless we enter it manually *after* an ambulance crew has been threatened assaulted.

Needless to say, one such report has been sent to central office.

I later found out that the patient was addicted to crack cocaine—which explains a lot.

RETURN OF PAVLOV'S EMT

Last night we picked up an alcoholic who is HIV positive. I (still) have no real fear of HIV patients, even when they are bleeding a bit and this patient was not (although they had wet themselves). The only problem is that I seem to have turned into one of Pavlov's dogs. When we found out the patient was HIV positive my stomach churned as if I were back on the PEP. It was really rather strange because it wasn't fear (I'll only have that when I'm due for my HIV test) but instead something more . . . biological.

The son of the patient was extremely embarrassed at the antics of his parent, and my crewmate spent some time making sure that he was alright.

NAUGHTY?

Is it naughty to take someone to hospital, who doesn't really need to go, just in order to get a fry-up breakfast there?

It's a lot simpler to take everyone to hospital whether they need it or not. It means that I have to do less paperwork, the patient feels validated and it means that if I'm missing something nasty (which is likely to happen at 6 a.m.) *then the hospital has a chance to catch it.*

TOO DARN BUSY

I am extremely busy at the moment; I'm often posting from my PDA (Personal Digital Assistant) and mobile phone. I should be catching up with stuff on Friday (including answering all those comments people have left).

Got some blood results (post PEP stuff), seems my white cell count is still going down. I think they have a life-span of 120 days, so it might get lower before it gets better. Still, it gives me an excuse to see the rather pretty occupational health nurse.

Today we did the usual of little old ladies who

feel unwell calling their GP and the GP calling us to take them to hospital because they are too busy to drag their arses out of their office to visit sick people. On the radio it seems that lots of people are dropping dead—the weather is quite a bit warmer (24°C) so the old are placed under a bit more physiological stress.

I have a hundred and one things to do, and no time to do it—simple stuff like paying bills can be incredibly hard when you are single and a shift worker.

And I think I'm moaning too much . . .

I'm off to bed now. Goodnight all.

HOW NOT TO STOP A STOLEN CAR

So damn tired . . .

I'm currently at that point where I wonder whether I am hungry enough to cook dinner before I go to sleep. Which biological urge will win out?

Today, our Control wanted us to go to an emergency call when we were the other side of the Thames—I rather politely asked them if we were the nearest motor as we weren't actually a boat, the reply was, 'Yes, do you have your water wings?'. So we ended up going a couple of miles out of our way to cross the river.

The call was a faint, probably from the heat that is roasting London at the moment—at least the women are wearing revealing clothes, which makes our job of cruising through the streets a bit more enjoyable.

Picked up two psychiatric drug-using patients in a row who were drunk and lying in the road perhaps 500 yards away from each other. Some children were poking one with a stick . . .

Then there was the 51-year-old 4-foot-4 Asian grandmother who, upon seeing her husband's car being stolen jumped on the back and hung onto the rear windscreen wiper. She was flung off and, thankfully, not seriously hurt—mainly bruising and gravel rash. Unfortunately, the car that was stolen also contained her house keys and bank books. The A&E was so busy they had to put her out in the waiting room—something that annoyed me no end, especially as the nurse that put her out there had annoyed me earlier in the day by suggesting that I didn't know what the symptoms of bulimia were.

Now to eat/sleep . . . then lather/rinse/repeat tomorrow.

☕ SUNDAY

Sunday alone in my flat, no work, no stress, some decent stuff on telly = Good.

No chocolate in the fridge, uniform to be ironed, work tomorrow = Bad.

Phone call from Occupational Health telling me my blood values are back to normal = Excellent (only HIV/hep test to go now).

🚑 EIGHT . . . NINE DOWN

Our complex is EIGHT ambulances short today, so it comes as no surprise that we are running around like the proverbial blue-arsed fly. Control keeps broadcasting jobs for which they have no ambulances, this means that a lot of crews are more unhappy than usual, as Control hassles us about 'greening up' quicker. It doesn't bother me, if I'm busy doing jobs it makes the shift go quicker.

As I'm typing this an ambulance has had a blow-out on the fast lane of the A102—a very busy road. The crew are alright, but it means we are now nine ambulances down for the next 2 hours at least.

The jobs I've been doing are the usual Monday morning sort of stuff: 97-year-old women having heart attacks, 10-year-old boys with cut heads (a rather impressive 3-inch cut, mind you) and 88-year-old men from nursing homes who have 'high blood pressure' (they invariably have a better blood pressure than I do).

Now some silly sod has stabbed himself in the stomach with a pair of scissors.

🚑 HEALTH COPYRIGHT

I've been on a 'Guidelines' course. Essentially, this is a course that tells us that we are already doing the right thing; it also introduces us to a book with our new treatment guidelines. It takes 2 days and tomorrow will include learning about child abuse (do we have to bring our own child?). So far the course has been a trainer telling us that this course changes nothing, and we are to continue doing what we are doing at the moment. At least the days are short, 8 a.m. 'til 2 p.m. At the start of every Powerpoint presentation is the same definition of 'Clinical Governance'.

We had to write our own scenarios then swapped them around to other groups (this is a really easy teaching technique, since you don't have to plan anything). There was also a chat about how our complaints to compliments ratio is about 50/50, and that most of the complaints are because of 'staff attitude'. So far I have had no complaints, and no compliments—I'm a strong believer of flying under the radar.

However there is a problem—the Guidelines book we should be getting is version 3.0, but the book we are actually getting is version 2.2.

The reason for this?

Copyright!

It seems that the LAS wants to change a few bits to make it more relevant to London. But because the organisation that wrote it maintains the copyright it can't be changed for us. Lawrence Lessig's 'Free Culture' states that you get value added when others can build on your work. This is a perfect example of this principle.

So, the people of London are not getting the best clinical care because of copyright.

Clinical Governance is about getting the best care to the public, so it's a bit of a mixed message.

VENUS TRANSIT

There is a Transit of Venus today—all these special astronomical phenomenon remind me of the eclipse we had in the summer of 1999 . . .

(Cue wobbly flashback video effects)

I was working in A&E at the time of the eclipse and thought that there would be no way I'd get to see it. Like all A&E departments this place had no windows and could be perhaps best described as a bunker.

Today, however, the department was empty for the first time in living memory. Normally by that time of the day we would be packed full, but today . . . not a soul. One person had been in earlier with a painful foot, but there wasn't the normal 'trolleys in the corridor' effect that was normal for that time of day.

We learned that day that CT (computed tomography) films make excellent sunglasses.

So, the whole department stood outside on the grass staring at the sun slowly disappearing—very spooky, and one of the few strong memories I have from that long ago. I suspect that many of the wards were empty as well: there was a procession of people wearing dressing gowns and holding tight to their drip stands wandering around the hospital grounds.

As soon as the eclipse finished we immediately had two cardiac arrests brought in by ambulance, it was as if they had waited until after the eclipse before deciding to keel over dead . . .

Life also tends to be a bit quiet around FA cup finals, royal marriages and important soap storylines.

NOT ALL BAD

I often carry a camera around with me. I was talking to some kids recently—they were happy little buggers, enjoying the sunshine on a lazy Sunday.

It's not all bad this job.

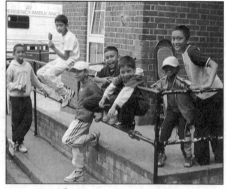

This picture still makes me smile.

Some calls are a pain in the arse, not because anyone is particularly ill, but instead because you can see complaints coming in, and there being a high possibility of losing your job.

Tonight was a case in point. We got called to a wedding reception where the bride had collapsed; a quick history revealed MS (multiple sclerosis), and that it was likely that this was the cause of the collapse. Unfortunately, the patient and the patient's new husband were adamant that she wasn't going to go to hospital, particularly the hospital that was nearest. Things were not helped because they had called an ambulance for an aunt who had collapsed, but had cancelled it before it had arrived because it was 'taking too long'.

While we were getting a history from the patient, the new husband was generally acting like an arse: he was questioning everything that we did, interfering with our talking to the patient and generally getting in the way. We managed to get rid of him for a short period and the rest of the family came over to us and apologised for his behaviour.

Luckily, the patient's hotel was next door to the hospital so, after 45 minutes of persuasion, I managed to get the patient to agree for us to take her towards the hotel, and if she felt better then we could, in good conscience leave her there. En route I called up on the radio, and arranged for the duty officer to meet us at the hotel. He did and the responsibility of leaving her without treatment now fell on his shoulders (thus, saving our jobs should anything go horribly wrong).

I know MS is a horrible disease. I know it isn't

fair that it would strike on your wedding day, and I can understand why you might not want to go to hospital . . . but if you can't move half of your body, then please understand why the ambulance people might be a bit unhappy to leave you lying in the middle of the street.

It then all kicked off in the Hackney/Homerton area. There was a big fight in a pub, with everything in it being smashed—multiple casualties with various head and facial injuries from flying bottles and broken glass. We were first on scene, and I needed to call up to let Control know that at least another three ambulances were needed. At least it gave me a chance to practice my '5-second triage' skills. None of the drunks there were particularly aggressive, but there was a ton of police there pulling me from one casualty to another around the pub, and even 300 yards up the street. This was just a taste of what was to come as another pub was attacked and it basically overloaded our resources. It got so busy that our Duty Officer was transporting severe asthmatic attacks in his car (and he doesn't carry much more than a defibrillator and oxygen) and Control was holding 35 calls across the area. That is, 35 calls at 3 o'clock in the morning. That'll teach me to wonder if it will be busy in a previous post.

Tomorrow England play their first 'Euro 2004' match—Alcohol + Patriotism + Recent History (we are playing the French) + Me working = Recipe for disaster

Watch this space . . .

I never got a complaint from that job, although for some time I was holding my breath about it.

🚑 KICK OFF

Well it looks like I was right, the nice weather with people in the pubs from an early hour, coupled with England losing 2–1 in the football has led to what can, in best tabloid fashion, be described as 'an orgy of violence'.

It started out with a couple of 'glassings', which we have been getting over our vehicle computer screens as 'stabbing to the head' for some reason.

A couple more assaults, including one who was set upon by a number of drunks who were intent on stealing his car. Luckily he was not too badly injured—more shook up. Other crews were 'blueing' in a number of assaults, including at least one stab victim.

The police were running from call to call, and once more there are not enough ambulances to deal with the large number of calls we have been receiving. Our Duty Officer has been telling crews that we should be wearing our stab-vests constantly—but he isn't the one who has to lug a 20-stone unconscious patient down four flights of stairs in this heat . . .

Good job I'm not searching for a quiet life.

I am, however, off to bed now.

🚑 ONLY ONE STABBING

For the first night in ages it has been reasonably quiet on the streets of East London—only one stabbing and that was to the patient's arse . . .

However, while adults are no doubt nursing hangovers the children are out causing mischief.

The first two calls we got yesterday were to kids (8 and 10 years old) who had been hit by cars. The first was a 'classic': child running out towards an ice-cream van. He was alright apart from a broken right ankle. No sooner than he was safely ensconced in hospital than we find ourselves dealing with a child who has run out in front of a car (in the absence of an ice-cream van) and has broken his *left* ankle.

Tie in a hyperventilating adult, a 14-year-old with hay-fever and a drunken Colles' fracture and you have a pretty good night.

We had one serious job, someone who had a CVA (a CVA is a 'stroke') on a train. The CVA wasn't so much the problem as the extrication of the patient, who couldn't move, and yet was combative with his unaffected side. To start off, the space between the seats on the train was not large enough to allow our carry chair to pass. The man was large and heavy so we basically had to manhandle him (in a very undignified manner) through some connecting doors and out onto the platform. The train station has a big flight of stairs towards street-level and only one lift, and the lift was not on the platform we were on. It would have been unsafe to carry this man up the stairs because of his weight and combativeness. In a rare spark of genius I realised that if we waited for a district line train we could carry him through the train onto the other platform. We 'blued' him into hospital as his pulse-rate was 40 (should be 60–100).

When I went to see the patient later in hospital he had started to regain his speech and wasn't confused. He was about to go for a CT scan so, with a bit of luck, he might make a good recovery . . .

This is just another part of the job that I like—that sometimes I have to out-think problems. I can't see me doing this in an office job.

🚑 GOOD SHOTS

There is something that I've learned over many years of health-care work. When you are lifting little old ladies with senile dementia, they will sometimes grab you by the testicles.

And squeeze . . .

This hurts.

I swear, the greater the degree of dementia, the greater the accuracy and the stronger the grip.

And for the love of all that is holy . . .

Don't drop them.

That hurts even more . . .

🚑 ETHNIC DRESS

When I went to the Clap Clinic for my HIV test, I was referred to a 'Health Adviser', which is a new name for Counsellor. I am, as regular readers may appreciate, a fairly simple, pragmatic person: within hours of my HIV exposure I was aware of transmission rates, odds of infection and the rates of death caused by electrocution (1 in 5 000) and shooting in America (1 in 2 500). So, to be honest, counselling was the last thing I needed.

I did a counselling course when I was a nurse, and it did nothing to disabuse me of the notion that all counsellors are hippies who consider themselves 'worthy'.

She asked me a load of questions about how I would cope if I were to be found HIV positive (answer: get over it), and cautioned me not to tell anyone I was testing, unless I was happy for them to know the result (answer: the whole world could know—if they read this site). There was some other stuff that is just too dull for words, and definitely to dull to read.

The thing that amused me the most, however, was not that the 'Advice Room' had the only comfy chairs in the place but that the counsellor was wearing a sari (the Indian dress). In and of itself not unusual, except that the woman wearing it was 'whiter' than me.

I'm well used to 'white' women wearing various Muslim dresses—it's a religion after all, but as far as I'm aware a sari is a cultural thing. I'm guessing that in her 'equal-opportunities, worthy, multicultural' world that she is proving how non-racist she is. This is handy because to be honest out of the 20 or more people at the clinic I was in a race/culture minority of one. Not a problem, I know Newham well . . . it's very diverse but, I wonder if Asian people would be impressed or nonplussed by her wearing a traditional Indian dress?

Maybe I should start wearing nothing but a Papuan penis sheath?

The HIV test result should be received by the 28th . . .

I've tried as hard as possible to make this sound as non-racist as possible—at no point have I meant to cause offence. I hate no 'race' more than another—I hate them *all*.

'I hate them all'—a philosophy to live by.

Our second call of the day was to an address where the elderly woman who lived there was believed deceased—the neighbours had called the police, and the police had called us. What this often turns into is us struggling to gain entry to the house, normally resulting in an injury to me, only to find someone who has been dead for some time.

We rolled up to the house and met with the neighbours who led us around to the back garden where, peering through the rear window, we could see the old woman sitting in her chair looking pale, still . . . and very dead.

Simultaneously, my crewmate and I jumped back in shock as we saw her take a breath!

She was breathing about six times a minute, and surely didn't have much longer left to live—I rushed around the front and kicked in the front door (in one hit—something I've never managed before) and we got her out to the ambulance in double-time. We quickly decided that it would be wrong to 'stay and play', instead opting to ventilate her via 'Ambubag' and to monitor her cardiac rhythm and her pulse (which was strong and regular).

The hospital had a team standing by, as we had notified them of the patient on leaving the scene. The transport time to hospital was about 2 minutes, and on arrival the A&E team leaped into action, intubating and ventilating her, gaining venous access and running the various blood tests. Family members were contacted and plans for her treatment were drawn up. At no time did I feel that this 88-year-old woman was receiving anything other than the best treatment possible.

We cleaned the ambulance and restocked before going on to our next job; each time we returned to the hospital we popped our head into the Resus' room to check how she was doing; there were plans to CT scan her head and to move her to ITU (intensive treatment unit). The family arrived and after some discussion it was decided that the best care for her was going to be palliative (that is to make her comfortable, but not to do any invasive procedures and to allow her to die). This was, I feel, the right course of action—the lack of oxygen would make any survival short and probably result in serious brain damage.

It has been a very long time since I've felt a great deal of sympathy towards someone, but this was one patient that I did actually care about, and not just because I'm soft on 'little old ladies'. She had little chance of recovery, but we hoped for it anyway. She fought for her life, and had probably been doing that for the whole of the night. Because of our actions, and the actions of the hospital team, she wasn't going to die alone, and she wasn't going to die without her family saying a final goodbye to her.

It's a small victory, but sometimes those are the only ones you get.

RIGHT TO 'LOAD AND GO'?

Yesterday we got a call to a 27-year-old male, diabetic having a fit. It was only 4–5 miles away, but travelling through Newham on a Saturday afternoon is always slow business—this was compounded by one of the roads which we use as a shortcut being closed for resurfacing. It took us 14 minutes to travel those 4 miles. Then it was up five flights of stairs into a flat where the first thing we could hear was hysterical sobbing. As I've mentioned before it's one of those sounds you know means trouble.

Squeezing past a large bed we entered the bedroom to find a First Responder 'bagging' the young man, who was lying motionless on the floor. Sitting on the bed wailing, was a young woman who we discovered later to be his fiancée. The patient was connected to one of our cardiac monitors and it was showing sinus rhythm. Kneeling on the floor I did a quick pulse check—beat, beat, beat . . . then nothing, no pulse for 10 seconds. During the pulse check I was getting a history. Apparently the patient was an insulindependent diabetic, who had possibly been neglecting to take his insulin injections. He had become more agitated during the morning until he collapsed and started fitting after having an argument with his fiancée.

With a monitor showing an apparent sinus rhythm the patient was in 'pulseless electrical activity'—we can't 'shock' this rhythm so I started CPR. From out of his mouth flew some bloody saliva, straight towards my face, luckily impacting on my forehead rather than ending up being swallowed (I don't want to make *that* a habit).

One round of CPR (3 minutes later) and we got a pulse—the patient started 'cramping up', all his muscles had gone into spasm. A very quick blood sugar measurement reading showed 'HI' (a reading of over 32.0 mmols of sugar—the normal is 4–7 mmols). Immediately I started thinking of DKA (diabetic ketoacidosis)—a condition that occurs when blood sugar goes too high—a life-threatening condition that could explain his cardiac arrest. There was little that we could do on-scene as he needed immediate medical treatment beyond what we could provide.

With a 'Load and Go' order my crewmate set up the chair and the three of us dead-lifted him over the bed that was blocking the door and into the chair—I felt the familiar trickle of urine down my leg and looking at the patient he seemed to lose all colour. Another pulse check followed—his heart had stopped again.

I had to make a decision then: would we start CPR again only for him to continue this cycle of pulse/arrest, or do we make a run for the ambulance—all the time starving his brain of oxygenated blood—so that we could get him into hospital to correct the cause of his arrest?

I decided that we should 'run for it': if we got a pulse back it would be a purely temporary measure until his high blood sugar could be corrected. It was a very difficult removal—my back was spasming as we carried him down the five narrow, dark, winding flights of stairs and ran him across the 100 yards of pavement to our ambulance. Throwing him and his fiancée in the back of the ambulance we started the long run back to the nearest hospital. For 10 minutes I did CPR in the back of the ambulance while my crewmate tried his best to get through the exceptionally busy traffic—stopping and starting, swerving across the road, over pavements; he drove to the limit.

Throughout transport the only rhythm we had was 'asystole', which is when the heart isn't beating at all. With our First Responder 'bagging' him and myself doing CPR we were doing all we could to support his life. During the transport the fiancée told us that he had had a previous arrest when he had stopped taking his insulin, but that he had, obviously, recovered.

Rolling up to the hospital we were met by the 'Arrest Team'—senior doctors from across the hospital. They descended on the patient, trying to get IV access, a secure airway and running diagnostic checks. It seemed, however, that the team leader didn't want to listen to our handover. I was later told that he was concerned about getting the audit times right. The first thing he said was 'the patient is biting on the airway' suggesting that the patient wasn't actually in cardiac arrest— because he hadn't listened to my handover he didn't know about the cramping episode earlier. The hospital staff did their own 'pulse check' and were confused about feeling a pulse (in a stressful situation doctors often feel their own pulse rather than the patient's). It was only after some time that I could actually give the team leader a complete handover that he paid attention to.

The team worked on him for over an hour. His blood tests showed that his potassium was a sky-high 7.5; this was probably the main cause of his arrest. It transpired that the patient had renal failure and the high potassium and high blood sugar probably meant that the normal biochemical reactions in the body were being interfered with, leading to his fitting and cardiac arrest.

One hour later the patient was declared dead.

His fiancée was distraught; the patient's parents had to travel 170 miles to the hospital and so it was necessary to tell them what had happened over the telephone—I can only imagine the drive down to London. The fiancée was convincing herself that it was her fault, that it was the argument that killed him, or that she should have recognised his symptoms of a high blood sugar before they became fatal. Both I and the nursing staff tried to console her, to tell her that it wasn't her fault—but would the parents blame her?

I was thinking, would he have survived if we had remained on scene longer? Was making a run for it the right decision, given that I knew we had to carry him down the stairs? Would he now be alive if he had lived in a house rather than a flat? Did he die because he was an 'angry young diabetic' who didn't want to comply with this treatment? He did have a history of taking an insulin overdose 2 weeks before.

It was a bad job, travel time was longer than it should have been, the flat was awkward to reach, it was difficult to remove the patient and the return journey to hospital was too long. It could have gone so much better. Although the patient might still have died it would have made us feel better. The job has left my crewmate and me a little depressed. Two deaths in as many days, one a 'victory' the other a real loss. I have today off so I'm going to relax and prepare for the joys of a night shift tomorrow.

One question for my medical readers: in the same situation would you 'Stay and Play', or would you 'Load and Go'?

I got a couple of replies to the question above when I originally posted it online. The best was a mnemonic that I have taken to heart: L.A.T.E.R

70

(Load And Treat En-Route). I don't want to fool around on scene with a sick person who needs to be in hospital.

THE CLIMAX DRAWS NEAR . . .

I'm feeling a bit fragile at the moment—these nights are really taking it out of me for some reason. I think the main thing that is getting me down is that I should be getting my HIV test result on Friday; as predicted, I haven't been worrying for the past 3 months (is it really that long ago?) but with the result due, it is sitting at the back of my mind nagging away. I'm confident that I'll test negative—even so I have the framework for two blog posts, one Negative, and one Positive.

Either way, I think I'll be having a drink or two after I get the result.

At the moment there is some confusion about how I actually get the result. The receptionist at the clinic didn't know if their telephone text messaging trial was still being used—I suspect that on Friday I'll hang around the ambulance station after the end of my last night-shift and then walk down to the clinic and get them to give me the result at 9 o'clock. It would be cruel to make me wait until after the weekend . . .

. . . So it'll probably happen, or they will have lost the sample or something similarly evil . . .

Tonight, the only job to really stick in my mind was a 'purple plus' (someone who has died and is beyond our help because of the amount of time they have been dead). It was an 85-year-old female who died, leaving behind her husband of nearly 70 years holding her hand. A very sad job, he was putting on a brave face, but I think later today it'll sink in. Hopefully, his son will be with him when it does.

So, dear readers, the next update to this blog (unless my leg drops off) will be after I get my HIV result; I'm not in a frame of mind to write anything legible at the moment (as I'm sure you have noticed). Hopefully, my next post will be Friday, but I'm a strong believer in the inherent evil of the Universe . . . so I'll talk to you on Monday.

🚑 NEGATIVE

Yep, the *title* says it all: the HIV test is negative, the syphilis test is negative and hepatitis tests are negative.

Needless to say I am so far beyond 'relieved' as to be numb with it all.

I spent the last 20 hours awake, first at work, then in the 'clap clinic' waiting room; I now think I deserve a deep relaxed sleep.

Goodnight, I'll write more when I wake up . . .
Posted at 11:13 a.m. local time.

🚑 FALLOUT

Well . . . I've had some sleep so I can now post in a slightly more focused fashion.

First off, thanks again to everyone who has shown support, either through the comments box, or via personal emails—it's all gratefully received. It looks like I'm going to have to find something else to die from now.

72

Tomorrow my brother and I shall be going for a nice relaxing drink, the first proper pub visit in over 3 months—there may well be a hangover involved.

I only had to wait 45 minutes at the 'clap clinic' for the test result—pretty hard to stay awake, but I think the emotional numbness that comes with exhaustion only helped me deal with the wait. The 'consultation' was over in less than 15 seconds: led into a room, asked to sit down and then told by a shaved-head counsellor that everything was fine. I didn't have a massive flood of emotion (possibly owing to the aforementioned exhaustion), but afterwards I sat on a stone outside the hospital, rang my mum and brother, text messaged my old crewmate and breathed a sigh of relief. (Old crewmate told me that I had to go and repopulate Newham—something I don't think I'll be doing quite yet . . .)

BOOZE OR POT?

I didn't sleep well last night—I think a total of an hour and a half—so if I'm a bit incoherent I'd like to register that as excuse number one. No real reason for the lack of sleep, it's a disadvantage of rotating shifts that every so often your body clock just throws up its hands in despair and goes to sulk behind the sofa, leaving you suffering insomnia and/or intense fatigue.

Last night was actually quite pleasant. The first job of the shift (at around 4 p.m.) was given as an 80-year-old male collapsed in the street. Making our way there we were beaten by not only the police and fast response car, but also by a Duty

Officer who had taken an interest in the job. It turned out to be a drunken Russian, actually in his early fifties who had decided to lie down and sleep it off in an alley. I suspect he was very surprised when he woke up to find himself surrounded by three police officers and four ambulance bods of various ranks. He was a pleasant enough fellow, who didn't speak a word of English, so to be on the safe side we loaded him onto the ambulance and took him to sunny Newham hospital. When we got there (and remember that this is around 5 p.m.) the crew before us, and the crew who followed us, both had people who were worse for wear for drink. Luckily for both our patient and the hospital a Russian nurse was working, so he could translate that the patient had indeed just drunk too much and would very much like to be left alone so he could go home. I'm always impressed by people who can speak another language, two people talking what sounds like utter gibberish, yet making complete sense to each other never fails to entertain.

When taking this gentleman to hospital I drove past six known drunks in the space of one street. Alcohol and alcoholism is a big blight on our society. On some shifts the only jobs we have are those influenced in some way by alcohol. Most assaults can be attributed to alcohol, frequent callers (sometimes six times in one day) are very often alcoholic, and the amount of 'collapse ?cause' jobs that turn out to be drunks is frankly astounding.

My personal view (and not the view of the LAS by any means) would be to prohibit alcohol, but legalise cannabis. Not only would it cut our workload by, at my estimate, 60–70%, but I've never had anyone high on cannabis try to hit me. Cannabis users are very rarely violent, tend to be generally easier to handle and seldom get loud and annoying. It's true that there are long-term health consequences, and that heavy 'stoners' can waste their life away, but the same holds true of alcohol and alcoholics.

On the rare occasions that I get called to someone on cannabis, it's normally because it is their first time and they feel 'dizzy'. Often a pat on the head, and an explanation that this is what is *supposed* to happen is enough to calm them down, and they will rarely require a trip to hospital. Because the intoxicant effects are fairly self limiting, people tend not to overdose on cannabis, unlike alcohol (which is why you find drunk people collapsed in the street).

There is one problem with the use of cannabis— I'm never sure what to call it in order to sound 'hip to the kids', the slang just befuddles me. Is it 'green', 'pot', 'hash', 'reefer' or 'draw'? At least alcohol is just 'booze'.

And now the government has made it even easier to get hold of alcohol with extended 'open hours'. Oh well . . .

🚐 TOO QUICK?

(What I'm going to post about might come across as being heartless, or myself being lazy—I don't think I'm either of them, but if you disagree with this post, as always, feel free to visit the blog and leave a comment)

75

Tonight we got called to a residential home for an 87-year-old female with 'difficulty in breathing'; once again it was way out of our area of coverage, but we made good time to get there. I've been to this home before, and it is one of the better ones I've visited; the residents are always clean, and appear well looked after. The care staff know their 'charges', and are always friendly, helpful and courteous towards ambulance crews.

I knew there was something wrong from the face of the member of staff who met us. She had a look of total concern, and I don't like to see that look on someone's face—it never bodes well. We went through the clean corridors and busy lounge of the home into one of the residents rooms. There were three nurses there, one of whom was crying (something I don't think I've ever seen before); lying in the bed was a little old lady who was extremely close to death. Her pulse was weak, and thready, something I could have guessed by the patient's colour. I very quickly told the staff that, yes, she was extremely ill and that she would have to go to hospital unless she had a 'Do Not Resuscitate' order. The staff said that it would be best to take her to hospital. We scooped her up, and her heart and breathing stopped in the lift to the ground floor.

I don't believe in a 'slow blue' (where CPR is performed by 'going through the motions' knowing that the patient will not survive and that the CPR is for the benefit of the relatives), so I started active, aggressive treatment while my crewmate drove us the 5 minutes to hospital. The patient remained in asystole (no heart activity at all) and on reaching hospital the doctors there declared her dead.

I may have previously mentioned the study that showed that 'out of 185 patients presenting with out of hospital asystole arrests, none survived to be discharged'. Both my crewmate and myself—and the hospital staff—knew that this patient had no chance of survival and that the reason we started CPR was because of our policy to commence resuscitation except in certain tightly defined circumstances.

If we had got there a minute later, the patient would already have died—in her bed surrounded by people that cared for her (although not her family) as opposed to being hoisted out onto a chair and then suffering the indignities of CPR in the back of an ambulance. While trying to resuscitate her during the transit to hospital I found myself looking into her dead blue eyes, apologising to her and hoping that she couldn't feel anything that I was doing to her.

I don't know if it is because I've had one and a half hours' sleep in the past 38, but it made me feel bad to put her through the indignity of pointless CPR. I know the policies are there to protect us (and members of the public), but sometimes I wish we could use some discretion.

Now I'll see if I can get some sleep.

I can still remember her sparkling blue eyes looking up at me.

🚐 FROM ONE EXTREME . . .

So, two nights ago I was dealing with death, people collapsing on the DLR (Docklands Light Railway), young men vomiting blood and looking like death warmed up, and women having miscarriages. Basically everyone I attended to on Wednesday night needed an ambulance.

Last night we had . . .

One patient with indigestion (for 2 years—FRU on scene when we got there as it was given as a 'chest pain').

One 'gone before arrival' (a drunk who phoned 999 complaining of a broken arm, but had wandered off before we got there).

One overdose 'acting violent', who also had gone before we turned up (driven to hospital by her brother).

One 'facial injury' (a woman slapped by her husband: no injury and she didn't want to go to hospital—her husband was taken away by the police).

One patient with ascites and chronic alcoholism, who was referred to hospital by the GP (could have travelled in her husband's car).

One call to a police station for an accused who had swallowed some drugs—he denied everything and the police doctor cleared his health.

And one patient with an arthritic knee . . .

The patient with an arthritic knee was a 70-year-old male who had called out his GP. Said GP had then diagnosed arthritis and decided that the patient needed hospital treatment. We got the call, and had to go out of the area we are supposed to be covering to pick the patient up. The booked hospital was even further out of our area—so much so it was in another sector.

When we got there the patient's son was present and as we loaded his father into the ambulance we were told that 'I'll follow up in the car'.

The look of sheer despair my crewmate gave me

78

had me in fits of laughter; thankfully, I was outside the ambulance so neither the patient (nor his son, who had gone to get the car) could see me.

There was no reason why the patient couldn't have been driven by his son, yet here we were, out of area, going even further out for someone who didn't need an ambulance.

Still, after the past few days it was nice to have a shift where no-one was actually 'ill', and so we could spend the shift in a fairly relaxed state.

We often get patients in this sort of situation. I've given up worrying about it, even if it does mean that an ambulance is tied up doing non-essential work. I just wonder how many people have died because of a delay getting an ambulance because we are forced to do these types of jobs.

DRIVING FOR THE LAS (FOR DUMMIES) PART 1 (ASSESSMENT)

When you apply for a job as ambulance personnel for the LAS, one of the things that they look for is that you are a competent driver. Therefore, as part of the interview process they throw you into the most run-down, barely working 14-seater lump of crap they can find, and tell you to drive around Earls Court. For those not from London, Earls Court is a congested area with fairly small streets, constant roadworks and the sort of people who think it is amusing to leap out in front of scared-looking interviewees on their driving assessment.

Before you see a vehicle you are given a piece of paper that tells you what the assessor is looking for, the crossing over of hands when steering is a big no-no, as is over-confidence (along with under-confidence), speeding, going too slow, incorrect use of gears, incorrect use of signalling and a myriad of other things you haven't worried about since you passed your driving test as a teenager.

When I first went for my driving assessment I noticed the 'over-confidence' bit, so I thought I'd be sure not to come across as too aggressive a driver. I was a model gentleman, I let people out of side turnings, allowed pedestrians to cross in front of me and didn't hassle people who were driving too slow: I failed my assessment for being 'under-confident'. 'Come back in 3 months' I was told.

Three months later and I was determined not to make the same mistake (an additional 3 months stuck in A&E nursing will make you ever so slightly determined). So, I got into the worst piece of crap in the fleet, and off we went. Leaving the yard I hit a kerb and about 200 yards down the road I did the same thing. 'Turn around and go back' I was told; I slunk back to the yard and vowed to do better in another 3 months.

Three months later, and I thought 'Sod it! I'm going to drive how I normally drive'. So I crossed my hands turning the wheel, sped up to stop signals, refused to let anyone out of a side road and drove as if I were driving my 1.0-litre Ford Fiesta.

I passed. Needless to say I was more than happy, and fairly skipped out of the yard that morning.

Of course this double failure didn't help my confidence when it came to the driving part of my training course.

All I can say is that I haven't run over any pedestrians, although I have reversed into some stationary objects.

80

🚐 DRIVING FOR THE LAS (FOR DUMMIES) PART 2 (TRAINING)

When you train to be an ambulance technician, you have to do 2 weeks of 'driving instruction' where you are split into groups of four, get given a 17-seater van that has been hired for you and you learn how to drive your ambulance using this equipment.

Perhaps the most important differences between an ambulance and the 17-seaters that we are given are that ambulances are automatic, while the 17-seaters are manual (I believe the American term is 'stick'), and that 17-seaters just don't 'feel' like an ambulance.

The training course consists of 2 days of fun, and the rest is chasing each other around the countryside at high speed.

The two days of fun include driving around a racing track, spinning around a skid-pan and swerving around traffic cones at high speed—both forward and in reverse.

Then, for the next 2 weeks, you learn some theory in the classroom, such as the 'limit point' and the forces that act on a vehicle (and why sometimes speeding up when you are losing control is a good thing). The rest of the time is spent driving at high speed around the countryside, making sure that you have the correct gear, speed and suchlike for high-speed cornering.

There are a few things that make this training course less than effective: the first is that as the *London* Ambulance Service, it is extremely rare that you find yourself driving in the countryside, it is also rare that you drive at any speed above

40 m.p.h. and, as mentioned earlier, ambulances are automatic vehicles and as such don't have gears.

I drove an actual, real ambulance a grand total of once during training. I sat in the driver's seat, pointed to the lever in the middle of the floor and said, 'what's that, and where is the clutch pedal?'

Luckily for me learning to drive an automatic is pretty easy.

At no point during the driving course did we drive on 'blue lights and sirens'—something that may have caused my first RTA.

(Insert wobbly flashback special effect here . . .)
The first day out on the road out of training school went well. I was attending (A&E nurse for some years) and my crewmate was driving (his previous job? 'Man and Van'—driving a removal van around London doing odd jobs). So the driving went well, as did the attending (dealing with sick people). The next day our roles were swapped, I warned our supervisor that I'd never really driven an ambulance before, but he said that we'd be fine if we worked like yesterday.

So, on my first emergency job, blue lights went on, sirens went on and people started moving out the way—it was then that I realised that you can't fit a 7-foot-2-wide ambulance through a gap made by two cars which is only 6 feet and 6 inches wide. This was the first time (and hopefully the only time) I've been sworn at by a boss, although to be fair, the only time I think I've deserved it. I learned how to fill in accident forms that day . . . and how to judge distances a bit better. (An ambulance is wider, longer and taller than a 1.0-litre Ford Fiesta.)

Soon my training came to an end and I was thrown into the world of emergency driving in Newham . . .

(End wobbly flashback sequence, cue end title 'To Be Continued . . .')

The boss who swore at me was right though. Even now I think that this is why I like the ambulance service over nursing. With nursing the boss would call you into the office to discuss your 'problem', and how I might 'reflect on what happened'. So for me, being sworn at was a breath of fresh air.

DRIVING FOR THE LAS (FOR DUMMIES) PART 3 (THE REAL DEAL)

After the assessment, the training and the first time racing around the streets of London being sworn at, you finally end up on your own, in a new part of town where you are expected to get to emergency calls in 8 minutes.

I got posted to Newham, which is a 10-minute drive from where I live; unfortunately, I'd never driven there and my navigation was awful. When I told my new workmates where I lived they thought, 'Good someone who knows the area' (and just after that they probably thought, 'If he lives *there* I wonder if he'll steal my car?'). This was before the days of satellite tracking where you just have to follow the dulcet tones of the computer (sometimes in Danish if some bright spark has reprogrammed the computer); in those days you had a mapbook and were expected to get on with it.

Gradually, you get to know the streets, where the regulars live, the pubs that are 'trouble' and where the 6-feet 6-inch width restrictions are. You then have to counter every threat the 'natives' throw at you.

For example, I might be driving a big white (or bright yellow) van, covered with flashing lights and 'ambulance' written on the side, occasionally—if I feel like pushing out the boat—I'll even have the sirens going. You might expect people to get out of the way; instead, pedestrians will be drawn to run out in front of you, like particularly dim-witted moths to a flame. People in cars will suddenly develop selective blindness, and idiots with Drum 'n' 'Bass pounding out from stereos worth more than their car will argue that I should make way for them.

Drivers will pull out from side streets in front of you, and as for the bizarre ideas some people have as to the best way to clear a path for us (jump on the brakes, swerve in front of us, sit there and panic), well, it's a good job we often don't have far to travel.

However, there are benefits to driving an ambulance: driving on the wrong side of the road (at a top speed of 20 m.p.h. mind you) still makes me happy, driving over kerbs is often a giggle, and let's face it, who wouldn't like to treat red lights as a 'Give Way'?

Despite popular belief, we don't actually go that fast—we can't, we never know when some young mother is going to push her baby buggy out in front of us. At best I think we have a maximum speed of 40 m.p.h., not only for our safety and the safety of other people, but purely because the worn-out ambulances that we drive have an acceleration that would embarrass a milk float, and a top speed of ...oh ... about 42 m.p.h.

told to meet with the Police and Fire Service at an RVP (meeting point). It turns out that some animal liberation types have taken offence to this company (rumour being they are supplying concrete to a new animal testing laboratory) and have sent some deactivated incendiary devices to various branches in order to scare them. Today, in three of the offices across London, some 'suspicious packages' had turned up and we were being sent to cover the defusing of one of these devices. Two ambulances, one Duty Officer, three fire engines and countless police were there, standing around the now evacuated offices.

Our Duty Officer started allocating 'Major Incident' roles to everyone. I don't think he was best pleased when I asked him why, when major incidents are designed to deal with multiple casualties, we needed to play that game when the only person in any danger in the now deserted office was the bomb disposal officer.

He sent me to arrange the parking of the emergency vehicles. We were soon stood down, however, when it was discovered that the 'device' was actually a packet of envelopes.

The next call was to two brothers who had fought over possession of a bong, with one brother trying to sell it to a third brother. Both we and the police were sent; when we got there both brothers had calmed down and there were no serious injuries. One policeman was confused about what a bong was used for, until I explained that it was 'drug paraphernalia'. One of the brothers told the policeman that he was selling it because he didn't use it—he much preferred smoking his cannabis in a spliff.

Luckily for him the policeman ignored this massive blunder (and me collapsing in tears of laughter at this idiot essentially confessing his drug habits).

Our next interesting job was to a man in Docklands who had a head injury caused by trying to avoid an attacking seagull. It turns out that there is a seagull living there who likes to dive-bomb people passing by. This man had ducked the avian attack, then tripped and fell flat on his face, knocking himself out. He had only minor facial injuries, but the loss of consciousness will mean a short stay in hospital being watched. My old crewmate suggested that he sell his story to the newspapers.

The rest of our jobs were rather boring after this early excitement.

SHOULDN'T YOU BE DEAD?

One of the things that will constantly amaze me is that some people will drop dead at the drop of a hat (so to speak), while others will survive injuries that would kill us mere mortals.

Today was a case in point: we got called to a 39-year-old female who'd been hit on the head by a brick that had fallen *seven* floors. We turned up at the location fully expecting to see someone with less of their brains inside their head than would be considered healthy. Instead, the woman was sitting in a chair (having had a C-spine collar applied) with her head supported by a BASICS doctor (a doctor who volunteers to respond to calls in the community).

This woman, who should have been dead, had a 1-inch cut on the top of her head.

. . . And that was it.

The brick had hit her on the head, then had hit the floor with such force that it had shattered. Yet, here she was with no injury other than complaining of the cut being painful. There was no loss of consciousness, but we treated her as if she had a neck injury, purely because of the 'mechanism of injury'. It's been a while since I've had to do a 'standing take-down' (where you get a standing patient onto a spinal board by placing it against their back and laying it flat with them on it) but it all went smoothly, the doctor travelled with us and was a pleasure to work with.

Although she was 39 the woman actually looked like she was in her early twenties—perhaps she has some witchy super powers? Either way she was discharged later in the day.

She was exceptionally lucky—if you can call getting beaned by a brick 'lucky'.

🚐 CRUNCH . . . CRUNCH . . . CRUNCH . . . MASKED SYMPTOMS

I discovered yet another reason to avoid alcohol, namely that it can mask the symptoms of otherwise obvious illnesses and injuries.

We got called to a 60-year-old man who had fallen in the street: as it was 2 a.m. we could guess that alcohol was involved. When we arrived on scene the patient was standing against a wall very much the worse for drink. Admitting he was an alcoholic he told us that he had tripped over and now his right leg hurt. While he was standing there I gave him a quick examination, he had no bony tenderness and was able to bear his weight on his leg. He could feel his toes wriggling in his shoe and there was no obvious deformity to the leg. We helped him walk the few steps to the ambulance, but he was unable to manage the stairs at the back of the ambulance so we put him in our carry chair and lifted him into the ambulance. Further examination showed little else of note; his pulse was a tad on the high side but otherwise his blood pressure and other observations were well within normal limits.

We transported him to hospital, where the nurse gave him a quick examination, essentially repeating the examination I'd given him in the field, and she sent him out to the waiting room.

When we returned to the hospital a little later we were told that he had a fractured neck of femur—essentially he'd broken his hip.

He was so drunk that he felt little pain, and for various reasons none of the normal signs of a broken hip were present. Luckily, I'd documented that I'd examined for the possibility of this type of fracture and found negative signs all the way along, so should he complain (which I doubt he would do) both I and the admitting nurse would be covered.

So . . . don't drink, or you may find yourself walking around on a broken leg.

Now I'm off to sleep. Two very long night shifts and I'm ready to collapse.

It's one of the main differences between A&E nursing and ambulance work—in an A&E department you have good lights, can undress the patient and can put them on an examination table. In ambulance work you can find yourself down dark, unlit streets, in the rain and with the patient lodged under a car. I did feel a little bad about this patient, mind you . . .

🚐 AN EXCELLENT BAD DAY

Have you noticed how much I talk about being tired or needing sleep? The benefits of shift work . . .

First off, I'm bloody knackered, frazzled, chin-strapped, and generally tired. If I ramble just poke me in the ribs with a stick.

Today was both bloody awful and rather good fun, which despite sounding like the ramblings of a madman is a perfectly sane way to describe today, although I'll be glad for it to be over.

The day started badly: I woke 3 minutes before my alarm was due to go off so I turned it off and woke for the second time 10 minutes before my shift was about to begin. I didn't get much sleep last night so I suspect my body overruled my brain to give me an extra 50 minutes of sleep.

Luckily, when I wake up with an adrenaline jolt like that I can get washed, dressed and speed through the streets of Newham like an Olympic sprinter on methamphetamine.

Turning up at the station I found out that my regular crewmate was ill, and instead a 'Team Leader' was being sent to work with me. Team Leaders are on the lowest rung of management: they are the people who are supposed to keep the troops in trim, and so spend considerable time moaning about the speed at which we get to jobs, and the poor quality of our paperwork. I'm of the

91

belief that if management don't know about me, I can't get in any trouble, so working with a new Team Leader was something I was less than happy with.

I had barely gotten to say hello to 'Team Leader' than we got our first call of the day, a 'Suspended' (cardiac arrest) a couple of miles from station. Manoeuvring a big yellow taxi through rush-hour traffic is no fun at the best of times, but as I was driving I gave it my best shot—we got to the scene shortly after our First Responder who was already bagging and giving CPR to an obese woman in her eighties. As we were in one of the new yellow ambulances I lowered the tail lift, got the trolley out and nearly ruptured myself lifting the patient onto the trolley bed. Rolling her out to the street, we got her on the tail lift and raising it, rolled her into the back of the ambulance. All that was left was for me to raise the tail lift the rest of the way and rush to hospital.

You may notice that I spent some time discussing the tail lift; this is because as I went to lift it, the hydraulics failed and it was stuck, sticking 7 feet out from the rear of the ambulance at a height of about 4 feet from the floor.

I gave it a kick, a shake and then resigned myself to manually lifting the bloody thing up, all while the crying relatives were watching me pumping the manual handle like an idiot. Finally, it was raised to the closed position, so I made my way rapidly to hospital while 'Team Leader' and 'First Responder' worked on the patient in the back. I'll not mention the road closure that forced me to make a painfully wide detour, but otherwise we reached the hospital with some speed where the woman was, unsurprisingly, declared deceased.

After a quick tidy-up of the back of the ambulance (which after a cardiac arrest always looks like a bomb site) we got a job to a 'unwell child'. The 15-month-old child was indeed unwell, although not life-threateningly so. The assessment was made harder by the mother having very poor English and the child having 'Development Delay', which encompasses a multitude of syndromes and genetic/biological causes.

The next job was a transfer from the local maternity department to a maternity department in another county. This is a hospital that I had no idea how to get to (the details of why there was a need for transport are too boring to go into; also, I think I might say something about the mother I'd regret in the morning). I set our travel computer to give me directions to the hospital and we set off. The journey was supposed to be 9.8 miles, but after following the computer's directions to the letter we had travelled *37 miles* along rather crowded motorways.

We had taken 30 minutes longer than we had planned. It's the last time I trust that bloody machine. 'Team Leader' was not happy about the computer but we laughed it off.

The next job was a simple maternity which we drove into the London Hospital. This was fine until I managed to drive into another ambulance when trying to leave the hospital. No damage to my ambulance, and minor damage to the other, but as my first accident in over 18 months, it was obvious that it would happen when 'Team Leader' was sitting next to me . . .

Returning to fill in the accident paperwork,

Control asked us to attend to another call—this time it was an obese unconscious 70-year-old female. She was extremely heavy and, because of her 'floppiness', was a complete dead weight. Once more I nearly killed myself lifting her. All her body functions and observations were normal so it was a complete mystery why she was unconscious, although I could confirm that she had been incontinent of urine . . .

. . . after I put my arm in it.

All these problems throughout the day meant that we worked harder than we needed to—and yet, throughout the day we had a great time as we laughed and joked between patients and vowed never to work together again. I said that I'd take sick leave, saying I was 'stressed' and 'Team Leader' said she would make sure I got sent to the other side of London before she worked with me again.

And so, at the end of the shift we parted, laughing at the thought that it was possible we could be repeating the experience tomorrow.

I'm looking forward to that possibility.

'Team Leader' is still on our Complex and is still a good laugh. Thankfully, I haven't had to work with her again.

BROKEN AMBULANCES

One of the main problems with the LAS at the moment is the lack of vehicles. In the past this has come to mean that there are not enough staff to man the vehicles that we have, or fill the rota to maintain safe cover over our area. Lately, however,

94

we haven't had the vehicles physically present. At the moment, I am typing this from work and looking out the window at the fitters whose job it is to maintain the fleet in our area of London. There are 13 ambulances waiting to be fixed. There are three crews sitting on station unable to take any calls because their vehicles have broken down.

Someone has just visited us in the staff car (a nice little Corsa) and, on attempting to leave, its clutch has broken.

Today I took an ambulance from West Ham over to Poplar to replace a vehicle whose steering had broken. Two management brought over a spare vehicle from Newham for me to work on—a vehicle that had just had a broken rear suspension fixed.

Let me tell you, riding on an ambulance with no suspension is an 'interesting' experience—you get thrown around and the cupboards fly open spraying bandages and other, less soft, equipment around the cabin.

This 'fixed' ambulance lasted three jobs before the suspension died again and I was bouncing around the cabin. It also stalled if you closed the choke.

So now I'm sitting on station twiddling my thumbs, unable to continue my daily grind of ~~saving lives~~ picking up drunks.

The fleet is just falling to bits, the new Mercedes have faults developing around the 5 000 miles mark and the tail lifts are extremely temperamental (like my experience yesterday—they fail at the worst possible moment). The LAS needs a cash injection so that it can have a fleet of basic, but reliable ambulances, fully equipped and fully manned.

Things haven't changed much since I wrote this, although with a few extra vehicles the turnaround for crews without a vehicle is a bit better.

🚐 AN APOLOGY TO A&E DEPARTMENTS

I would suggest that a lot of the people who read this are doctors and nurses of one persuasion or another. I also guess that many of these readers have some experience of A&E departments.

So, as an EMT I wish to apologise.

I'm sorry that throughout the shift I will continue to bring fresh meat to the grinder, that is, I will be forced to transport patients from 'outside' into your department, where they will need to be looked after and assessed by your own good selves.

I'm sorry that I have to sometimes bring their relatives who will harass you about waiting times, the pain their relative is in and about why you are drinking that cup of coffee while their dearly beloved is 'at death's door'. I'm also sorry that sometimes I couldn't bring the only relative who can translate the patient's moaning and groaning into English, thus making assessment a thousand times easier.

I'm sorry for the dross that I bring to you: the cut fingers, the bellyaches and the spotty backs. I'm sorry that the primary health-care workers (the GPs) are often so useless as to be a liability. I'm sorry that you have to cope with the fallout that occurs because there are so few good GPs and you have to become the first point of call for coughs, colds and diarrhoea

I'm sorry that the schools don't teach basic health and first aid to their students, preferring to waste time on the history of glaciers or the solving of quadratic equations. This means that the population wouldn't know the difference between a minor cut and an arterial spurt if it jumped up and hit them over the head with a hammer, neither do they know which of these two injuries warrants a trip to the local Emergency Department.

I'm sorry that our communities where our Elders teach our Youngsters and the Youngsters listen no longer exists, resulting an influx of first-time mothers who think that when a baby vomits it is a precursor of death.

I'm sorry that the protocols and guidelines that we adhere to don't allow us to leave patients at home. In England at least, we have to transport to hospital. The government thinks that we cannot tell the difference between serious cases and the aforementioned cut finger.

I'm sorry that the police cannot look after drunks on a Friday night; they worry that they will choke to death in the cells, and so we get called. We have nowhere else to take them to but your department. Sorry.

I'm sorry that I bring in those serious cases 5 minutes before your shift finishes. If it's any consolation it's probably 5 minutes to the end of our shift that people decide to have their heart attacks, their amputations and their dissecting aortic aneurysms. Like you, this means we get off late as well.

I'm sorry, but it's not my fault.

I wrote this in part because we do sometimes get dirty looks from A&E staff as we drag in the umpteenth drunkard of the shift. It's not my fault that the government made 999 so easy to dial.

Gillick competency is the ability of youngsters under the age of 16 to give informed consent for medical treatment. Essentially, we have to assess whether a child is competent enough to make decisions about their own body. This is, as you might guess, is an ethical minefield.

Back to work with the rather enjoyable 18:00–01:00 shift, where you tend to get lots of drunks, and very few *serious* cases that require me to do some actual work.

However, you do occasionally come across a job that is tricky, not because I worry about the patient's illness, but instead for reasons that to the non-ambulance person are hard to understand.

Our first job of the day was one of those very jobs. The call we were given was 13-year-old female with a dislocated knee. Nice and easy I hear you say, but lots of minor problems can build up to make a job less than ideal.

We arrived on scene and found a patient who had a rather obvious dislocated knee—just imagine your kneecap shifted 2 inches to the left, so much so that it casts a shadow on the rest of your leg. Simple enough to deal with: if you are feeling brave you can slide it back into place yourself, or go the more recommended route which is to take the patient into hospital and let the doctors fiddle with it.

Then the problems started piling up. To start with there were no adults present, just another (unrelated) teenager; neither the patient nor this other teenager were what you would exactly call brain surgeons. We are not supposed to deal with

98

children without an adult present, but what else can you do in those circumstances? The father had been called, but he was travelling from another hospital where he had been undergoing outpatient treatment. So we had to decide whether it was 'safe' for us to take the patient to hospital—we use 'Gillick competency', but it's always a bit of a gamble on our part.

The patient had fallen from her bunkbed so her friends (who had run off) had lifted her *back* onto the top bunk. She was screaming in pain (which is fair enough I suppose), and wouldn't let us near her. This little problem was solved by giving her a lot of Entonox (known to some people as 'laughing gas'). After enough of this stuff she started laughing and we essentially 'grabbed' her off the bed.

Then she refused to sit in the carry chair, but because we were upstairs she needed to go in it. After a *lot* of persuasion, and a lot of her screaming very close to our ears, we managed to get her to sit down; this had the rather excellent side-effect of popping the kneecap back in place.

This would normally mean that the amount of pain goes down by a lot, but this girl had a touch of 'hospital phobia' so she continued screaming. While screaming she was also arguing with the teenager who was with her, telling him that he needed to come to hospital with her but he was refusing because 'How am I gonna get back home?'. I must admit I really wanted to tell him to walk it, because the hospital was only about 1 000 yards away. Despite her pleading with him, he wasn't for budging. He set his burberry baseball cap square on his head and refused. I don't think she is going to be too happy at him next time she sees him.

Once that argument had run its course (and my crewmate and I managed to stop laughing), we had to get the patient downstairs—this was made more difficult by a sideboard that was in the upper hallway by the stairs. To counter this problem, we had to lift her completely over the banister. Luckily she was a lightweight, and my crewmate and I are—*cough*—both strapping, good-looking men.

We saw her later in hospital, having a plaster cast put on her leg, so that the kneecap wouldn't slip out of place. She was much happier and surrounded by her parents. She even managed to give us a smile, which, in the end, made the job worthwhile.

So, this is what we occasionally have to deal with, not so much the life-threatening stuff, but more the silly little things that can make an 'easy' job much trickier.

DRUNK AND DISORDERLY

We got called to a pub (which is always promising), to a 24-year-old female who was having 'difficulty breathing'. When we turned up at the pub, we were met by a man who, after letting us know he was a 'first aider', told us that she was fitting and that she had stopped breathing, but that mouth to mouth resuscitation had 'brought her back'.

Entering the pub we found the woman thrashing around on the floor. She wasn't having a fit, it was more like a temper tantrum. Throwing himself on top of her was her husband, who was reluctant to let us approach her. People in the pub told us that they had both been drinking heavily.

We near enough had to force the man off of his wife just so we could examine her properly, and it soon became apparent that she was just very, very drunk. Out of the corner of my eye I saw sudden movement and ducked quickly as the husband threw his wife's shoe at a man standing behind me. We decided that loading her onto the ambulance would be the best thing to do. The husband demanded to be let in, but we told him that we needed room to properly examine his wife. He banged on our windows twice, but then left, apparently running up the road—possibly as a result of him throwing a pint glass at another of the pub's customers. (This was very unwise of him, because half of Newham police force were 200 yards up the road dealing with an armed incident.)

By this time a second crew had turned up, as someone had called 999 and told our Control that the woman had stopped breathing. We stood them down, although, on reflection, they could have been of help keeping the woman on the trolley because she was still throwing herself around, refusing to lie still, and generally making life difficult. We managed to get a blood sugar, pulse and blood pressure (all of which were normal) but she refused to stay on the trolley and wouldn't sit on a chair—so we let her lie on the floor.

At times like these, I think I'd give my eye-teeth to be able to put people like her in a four-point restraint, but it's something we are not allowed to do.

Later, while I was driving to hospital, she made an attempt to leap out the back of the ambulance, and it was only the rugby skills of my crewmate that prevented her escaping under the wheels of a following car. The rugby tackle was all the more impressive given that my crewmate is 5-foot-nothing tall.

We finally managed to get the patient to hospital, where she threw her vomit bowl (with vomit) over the floor and tried to hit a nurse. Luckily I was standing behind her and grabbed her before she could damage any of the staff, or even a patient.

To cut a long story short, the nurses let her phone her sister to come and pick her up, and then kicked her out the department.

Two things about this job that bring a smile to my face: (1) one of her shoes is still lying in the gutter, where we picked her up from, and (2) her husband got out of prison today and, given his attitude and behaviour, he'll soon be back inside.

So, it's not just weekend nights we get the violent drunks, it's every damn night . . .

We are not taught how to restrain patients who might be violent but sometimes it is essential—for example, in the event of someone having a serious head injury and becoming violent. So, we have to make it up as we go along and hope that it turns out alright.

FAVOURITE JOB

The other night I had my favourite type of job, the type of job that meant I wasn't upset to be late leaving work.

People who are diabetic sometimes have very low blood sugar; this makes them confused, agitated and sleepy, and this can lead to unconsciousness and even death. Their blood sugar can become low for any number of reasons. Most often they have done more exercise than normal and not eaten enough to raise their blood sugar.

The treatment for this condition is to either give them sugar or an injection that 'frees up' some sugar that is stored in their liver.

Our patient last night normally controls her diabetes very well; so much so that her family had never seen her with a dangerously low blood sugar (the medical term for this is hypoglycaemia). They called us because she was acting confused and was unable to speak properly or stand upright. We arrived, and found out she was a diabetic; checking her blood sugar we got a reading of 1.6 mmols (the normal range for a diabetic is around 4.5–12.0 mmols)—this is very low and explained why she was losing consciousness.

The family were understandably upset, as they had never seen this before. They saw her slipping into a coma in front of our eyes, so we explained what was going on as I prepared the injection that would raise her blood sugar. I gave the injection (this injection is called glucagon) and waited for it to take effect, all the time reassuring the relatives.

Within 10 minutes she was up and talking, we then gave her some sugar jelly which raises the blood sugar some more. Soon she had made a full recovery, with her blood sugar reading 5.6 mmols. We gave her some carbohydrates (for 'slow-burn' energy) and left her in the care of her exceptionally happy family.

The reason why this is such an enjoyable type of job is that we are actually saving a life (for a change) with the treatment that we can give, and that the recovery is normally rapid, and always impressive. From unconsciousness to 100% fitness in the space of about 15 minutes really impresses onlookers . . . and it does our ego good to be praised every so often.

NOTTING HILL—*STABBY, STABBY*

Yesterday was the last day of the Notting Hill Carnival. The police are calling this year's carnival a success, with little reported crime, but I would tend to disagree: its just that the crimes all happened to people as they travelled home.

Our second call of the night started worryingly when Control told us that a male had been stabbed in Stratford shopping centre, and that he could still hear shouting in the background of the call. The stab vest went on and we made our way down there, meeting up with a lot of police officers trying to control a rather large crowd of post-carnival spectators.

We found a 15-year-old male lying on the floor, with a policeman holding some paper tissues over an upper abdominal stab wound. There was no external bleeding, and the patient was alert, calm and talking. He also had a small wound to his right leg, which again was not bleeding significantly. I ran through a primary survey (a very quick examination of the patient to rule out anything that is going to kill him in the next 5 minutes) and then concentrated on making sure his chest and lungs were not damaged. On clearing them I turned my concentration to the belly wound.

We don't like stab wounds: they can do a lot of damage leaving only a tiny entry wound. One stab wound can easily kill you, whether it is in the leg, the arm, the chest, or the belly. After my examination I decided that, although he needed exploratory surgery, he wasn't critically ill. There was a bit of 'something' poking out of the wound, I had no idea what it was (I initially thought it was part of the policeman's dressing) so I soaked one of our dressings in saline and applied it to the wound. We then got a phone call from what I took to be the HEMS road team (a doctor and paramedic) letting us know that they would be on scene in 12 minutes and that the patient should go to the Royal London Hospital. The problem with this is that the Royal London is some way further away than Newham, and that I knew that if the HEMS crew got on scene they would want to 'stay and play' securing IV (intravenous) lines, considering intubation and running a full examination on the roadside. In my opinion, having assessed the patient, his best option would be to go immediately to the nearest hospital and let the surgeons there deal with him.

So, we loaded the patient onto the ambulance and made a run to Newham Hospital which took us less than 5 minutes.

The result of which was the patient got to theatre, was 'packed' as he had a lacerated liver and gall bladder and is now in ITU for recovery.

I wonder if the HEMS crew will moan. I suspect they won't because around the corner was another young lad who had been stabbed in what later turned out to be a connected series of battles between two schools. The HEMS crew played around on scene with that patient before taking him to the Royal London Hospital (who really love their trauma jobs). There were then reports throughout the night of other crews picking up more teenagers injured during the fight. The patients were spread fairly evenly between the two hospitals, so no one department became overloaded.

A couple of things struck me as amusing, the first was that when we were about to leave for hospital the patient's girlfriend and cousin were fighting among themselves over who loved him more and should go to hospital with him. The patient's brother was also there and was fighting with police to get to the patient. He then vanished, and my prior experience would suggest that he was planning revenge and a counterattack.

While going to hospital, the patient's girlfriend was talking about the other lad who had been stabbed (apparently his name is 'Biggy G') and how it seemed that the fight had been planned at the carnival.

As always when I got to the hospital it seemed that the doctors weren't interested in my handover . . . on which I will post/moan more later.

As we were going to hospital another crew, this time in North London, were putting in a priority call to their local hospital. They had two young men (aged 19 and 20) who had been stabbed, luckily in a non-serious manner.

A night full of people getting stabbed. Just a coincidence that is the last night of Notting Hill? The media said that the carnival passed without serious incident. Either they were not looking very closely, or they decided not to report the violence around the capital.

106

Some jobs will just make you sad, and it's those that you'll find yourself carrying around with you for a time. It isn't always the death and horror that affects you, and you can be surprised by the things that haunt you.

We got a call to a block of flats, it was given as a 69-year-old female who was unresponsive and who had a history of schizophrenia. Her condition could be caused by any number of things, so you carry all the equipment up the flats as you never know what you are going to encounter.

We were met by the woman's husband who led us through to the bedroom where our patient lay. She was on the bed and was not talking to anyone; with one hand she was 'fidgeting' and plucking at her clothes. This was normal for her, and could be due to the antipsychotics she uses to treat her schizophrenia. Looking at her prescription sheet we found out that she was also a diet-controlled diabetic, but her blood sugar test showed a normal amount of sugar in the blood. The patient was unable to talk, and looked very scared. Was this episode related to her schizophrenia?

Our physical exam, however, showed a complete loss of function and muscle tone down the right side of her body; this led us to think that she had had a CVA, or stroke, and that this had affected her speech and muscle function. We rapidly removed her to hospital, and, to be honest, the job itself went like clockwork.

The thing that stays with you though, is her husband telling you that they have been married for 50 years, and for the last 20 of them he has stuck by her while she was suffering first from manic depression and then schizophrenia. To have stayed by her side while she was under the shadow of these illnesses shows true love. Every so often, during the transport to hospital, her husband had to wipe a tear from his eye; he was sitting holding his wife's hand, trying to provide some comfort to her and ease the scared expression on her face.

If she survives the stroke she will probably be permanently disabled and will require quite intensive care for the rest of her life.

I think her husband will continue to stand by her.

In unrelated news . . . I was so tired driving home this morning that I took the wrong turning to go home and went down the wrong street. Aren't you glad I'm looking after the health and well-being of people?

🚐 UPDATE ON LAST POSTING

Lots of people want to know what happened to the lady in my previous post, so tonight I spoke to the nurse who was looking after her.

The patient continued to be unable to talk, although (perhaps sadly) she could understand everything that was happening to her, and around her. She was also unable to use the entire right side of her body. It seems that the stroke was caused by an infarct (or clot) in her brain and not the more life-threatening cerebral bleed. She went to one of the better wards in the hospital after spending some time in the Resus' room, during which her husband constantly stayed by her bedside. The nurses looking after the pair of them felt a lot of sympathy towards them, and I think they all fell a little in love with the husband.

I mention that the nurses looked after the pair of them, because that is what good nurses do, they look after everyone *affected by the illness.*

Sometime later today or tomorrow she will have a CT scan of her brain to determine the extent of any infarct, and then she will start the long road to a hopeful recovery.

I used to work in a medical ward, and we would have a lot of stroke patients. Unfortunately, there is no magical medical treatment for a stroke once it has taken place; instead, it is a long gruelling slog through physiotherapy, speech therapy and occupational therapy. It can take months to recover some function, and many do not recover at all: they remain chair- or bed-bound and are discharged into a nursing/care home until they succumb to an infection that kills them.

Unfortunately, given the type and strength of the stroke this lady has had I would not hold much hope for a recovery. Miracles do sometimes happen, and I suspect that this entire woman's family will be praying for such a miracle.

🚐 TRICKY EXTRACTION

I think I've mentioned on more than one occasion how, when working in a hospital, the patients are often nicely 'packaged' ready for examination, this can often hide the trauma that the ambulance crew has gone through in getting the patient into hospital in such a condition.

My crewmate and I got called to a 'collapse', and we made good time getting there to be met by relatives of a 72-year-old female who had vomited altered blood (probably from a stomach ulcer) and had collapsed to the ground hyperventilating. The woman was around 20 stone in weight (280 pounds to the Americans in the audience). She was in a bungalow, so we had no stairs to get in our way, and the relatives were willing to be helpful. The patient was lying on the floor and had just finished an episode of hyperventilation (a panic attack).

Should have been a nice easy removal, even with the weight of the patient and reduced ability to walk. We had our carry-chair and after struggling a little to get the patient on it, we didn't expect any trouble.

Heh . . .

It turned out that the patient was an agoraphobic and hadn't left her house in 20 years . . .

Sweating profusely, the patient fought us the entire way out of the house; she grabbed at anything tied down, at door-frames and at the handrail she had installed in her house. Trying to get a sweaty 20-stone patient out of a house is tough enough without them fighting you the whole way.

We had explained that she needed to go to hospital, and she had logically agreed, but this didn't stop her panicking when we started to move her. When we finally managed to get her into the open air her panic rose to a dangerous level.

She was shaking, her eyes rolled back into her skull, sweat was pouring off of her and her thrashing about in the carry-chair got worse (if such a thing was possible). Both my crewmate and myself thought that she was going to have a heart attack; in fact, she had all the classic symptoms of a massive myocardial infarction (posh medical term for a heart attack). Then she started a strange screaming/moaning call that sounded completely unearthly. I could just see the next days newspaper headline, '*Ambulance Crew Scare Patient To Death!* '

All I could think about was to try and calm her down, so I tried using some hypnosis techniques that I just happen to know, which helped a little, but by then she was in such an agitated state that horse tranquillisers probably wouldn't have affected her.

We managed to get her into the ambulance, where we shut the doors very quickly and made as smooth a transport to hospital as possible. During the transport my crewmate and the patient's family worked constantly to calm the patient down, but they were only having a fairly limited success; every so often I would hear her moan in that alien fashion and my crewmate babbling at her to calm down.

When we got to the hospital, we nearly threw her off the ambulance into the A&E department; actually, she was so slicked with sweat we could have slid her off the trolley. She calmed down a bit once she was in hospital, which only made our exhausted faces seem over-dramatic to the nursing staff.

You never know what you are going to get in this job, but nine times out of ten it isn't the illness that surprises you, but the circumstances around the job.

I can't drive past that address without thinking about the trouble we had with that call.

We got called as a 'second crew' to an address. Sometimes, when a situation is beyond the capability of one crew to deal with, they will request another crew; normally this is because they have two patients, or the one patient that they have is too heavy for one crew to lift on their own.

We got the job as 'female giving apple to 7-day-old baby', which had us wondering . . .

As we turned up we saw the other ambulance and a police car. On entering the flat we saw two policemen standing in the corner, with a 5-foot 2-inch tall female paramedic *sitting* on a young woman (Patient Number 1); her crewmate was dealing with a male who had a nasty bite on his arm (Patient Number 2). The police were talking between themselves deciding what to do, as we got a quick briefing from the crew who was sitting on the woman.

It turned out that the woman (who had a previous mental illness episode), had given birth by Caesarean section 7 days earlier, and today had tried to feed the baby apple pie; she had then 'freaked' (note the professional medical terminology), shouting that the man wasn't her husband, and had attacked him. The ambulance crew had been called and, as they arrived, the woman had sunk her teeth into her husband's arm. The crew had fought the woman to—ahem— disengage her teeth, and this is why they were sitting on her. The police had been called, but were reluctant to do anything (I got the impression that they were a rather crap pair of coppers) and the second crew (us) had been called to deal with the husband (with new teeth-mark wound) and baby.

This woman was (brace yourself for more medical terms) 'completely bonkers', she had the rolling eyes, the delusional thoughts and the inability to communicate that separates the mildly strange from those who need immediate medication. It was actually quite sad to see this family come apart at the seams; the husband was shell-shocked, the wife was completely detached from reality and the police weren't being very helpful (which is unusual).

We got the husband and baby out of the house and into the back of our ambulance, and then returned to see the police (finally) manhandling the woman out of the house and into the back of the first ambulance. She was securely strapped down (although we don't have restraints, so she could have easily gotten free if she so desired); we had to lend the first crew a belt-strap as the one on their trolley was broken. The first crew then forewarned the hospital about what they were bringing in (violent schizophrenic female) and we all set off for the hospital.

We got there first and advised the nurse in charge that this was a 'real' warning and that security guards would be needed, along with the private 'psychiatric' room. It took her 20 minutes to arrange both, while the ambulance took less than 5 minutes to get to the hospital. So, while the secure room and security was being arranged this very disturbed woman was lying on the ambulance trolley . . . Not a good situation, and it made the job a lot harder than it should have been.

The husband was completely stunned; he had no

idea how to look after a baby and quite simply couldn't cope. Social services were informed, and the child was admitted to the paediatric ward for a while, until the husband could be taught how to look after a baby. The woman was sent to the local psychiatric unit for assessment and treatment; hopefully, this is a temporary condition brought on by childbirth (puerperal psychosis). The husband had his wound treated, and was sent home.

Oh, and the baby is a hermaphrodite.

There are jobs that you can recount around a dinner table (or at the pub) when people ask you what your job is like. This is one of those jobs, although for some reason people seem to prefer hearing about me being injured by little old ladies.

HOLY JOE'S

The London Ambulance Service doesn't just deal with emergency calls to people's houses, we also do hospital transfers—patients who go from hospital to hospital because the original hospital hasn't the expertise to deal with that person's medical problems. An example of this would be the transfer I recently did from Newham to the Royal London because Newham's CT scanner was broken, and the patient needed an emergency scan.

One of the regular places that we find ourselves transferring people to is St Joseph's Hospice, or as we call it Holy Joe's. Sometimes we will be picking up patients from one of the nearby hospitals, sometimes from the patient's own home. Its one of those jobs most of us don't mind doing. The patients are, by definition of needing hospice treatment, actually sick, and we are not so hard-hearted that we would begrudge an ambulance to someone who is ill. Then there is Holy Joe's itself . . .

Holy Joe's is a religious place, it used to be run by nuns, but now they are a bit few and far between. To be honest, I saw my first nun there yesterday, and she was picking her nose . . . But, you walk into the place and it just seems nice, it is clean, the staff are all friendly, the patients all seem happy and there is a really good social atmosphere there. I don't know if it is because of its ties to the religious orders (I hate all religions, but the best nursing homes always seem to have nuns running the place), but the hospice just seems to exude calm.

My crewmate and I had just transferred a terminally ill patient into Holy Joe's and were having a cup of tea in their tea bar (hot drinks are free to the LAS—another reason to love Holy Joe's). Sitting in this clean, comfortable area, we were watching the patients chat with relatives, staff and other patients, giving the place a real friendly atmosphere quite unlike anywhere in the NHS. It is very rare to see a doctor sitting down with a patient, chatting about nothing in particular and having a cup of tea with them. We both agreed that this has got to be one of the better places to see out the end of your days, and that it is a real shame that there are not more places like this.

It is a shame that in this increasingly 'technical/ evidence-based/audit/professional development/ governmental targets' style of health service, we seem to have forgotten that sometimes we simply, and honestly, need to care.

115

I went back there for the first time in 18 months. It's even better now. I'm thinking that the NHS should poach the board of directors and point them at some of our local hospitals.

ASSAULTED AND HAPPY ABOUT IT

I got assaulted yesterday, which made me smile . . .

We got called to 'Male collapsed outside park', which immediately set my 'drunk-o-detector' bleeping. This is the sort of call that is nine times out of ten, a drunk who has decided to have a sleep in a public place as opposed to going home. In a case like this we tend to wake them up, and get them to move on before another 'good Samaritan' calls us out again.

We woke him up, so he stood up and started moaning that we had woken him up. Both my crewmate and myself were actually being quite nice towards him—mainly because it was towards the end of our shift and being nasty to people takes energy that we just didn't have. Then he decided to take a swing at my crewmate, then he decided to have a swing at me . . . the next thing that I knew I had him in an armlock up against the side of the ambulance. My mate called on the radio for urgent police assistance, and the radio controller asked if we were both alright, to which my crewmate replied 'I'm alright, but my crewmate is restraining him'.

The police were quick to turn up, and I had just enough time to tell them that he was drunk and had taken a swing at us before he was under arrest and carted off to the local police station. It was

116

then I realised that in the struggle I'd managed to hit myself in the chest, right where I've got a broken rib. It was a bit painful. It had already gotten a whack from a heavy trolley yesterday, so I'm wondering if it will ever manage to heal.

I can tell you what went through my mind as I was pinning him to the ambulance: the first thing was 'Oops, I hope I haven't over-reacted', the next thought (about 5 seconds later) was, 'By the time I return to station and fill in the 'incident form' my shift will be over . . . Result!'. I'd imagined that, going by the speed that the police arrested him they were close to the end of their shift as well.

I'm just waiting for a Team Leader to read the incident form and call me into the office to ask if I need counselling . . .

A police friend of mine emailed me a couple of months later telling me that he had been in court providing evidence and the case before his was of a drunk assaulting an ambulance person. After a further description I could tell him that it was me who'd been assaulted. The drunk was found guilty, but had no penalty to pay as he was homeless. It would only have bothered me if he had actually connected with his punch.

🚐 DEAD BABIES

One of the jobs that we find ourselves going on (perhaps once or twice a day) is that of vaginal bleeding, in a woman who is around 8 weeks pregnant. This invariably turns out to be a miscarriage. Unfortunately, it is normal for the body to 'reject' a foetus that has no chance of developing into a full-term baby. I would suppose that this stops a woman from carrying to term an infant that would not survive outside the womb.

While dealing with such patients (some of whom have been trying to get pregnant for some time), I always try to be sympathetic, and explain that what is happening is not anyone's 'fault', and that it is a normal happening.

Because of the number of people we have with this problem, and the rate at which hospitals deal with them (when working in A&E we would have about 12–18 cases of this *every day*) we have all become a little blasé about it. We feel some sympathy, but deep down in our hearts, we know that there is nothing we can do, and that it is a good thing that this is happening now, rather than in 6 months' time. Nonetheless, we are worn down by the sheer numbers, and at the end of the day, perhaps we stop caring that these women are losing babies.

I have no intention of getting into the whole abortion argument, I've seen them done, don't like them and would rather have the whole thing stay out of my world view.

I first thought that it was just me, and that as a male I was not best placed to pass comment. However, after having a chat with some female colleagues, it seems that they feel the same way I do, that it is natural, and that it is not worth worrying about. But it worries me a little that I seem to have come to care so little for the dead babies.

There were two interesting jobs today. I'll tell you about one now and let you wait until tomorrow for the other one.

We got called to the very common 'Male Drunk—Police on scene', I'll not moan about how often we get called to this type of job, you've heard it all before . . .

We arrived on scene and were met by a policeman who first apologised before leading us to a man who was approximately 30 years old. The man was obviously drunk, and my crewmate told me that he smelt heavily of alcohol; along his arms were the scars of a 'cutter'—something else we are seeing more and more of these days. The policeman told us that the patient was refusing to give his name or medical details, only that he was called 'John'.

We approached 'John' and he agreed to come to hospital with us. I got him into the back of the ambulance and he refused to let me touch him, so I couldn't do my usual battery of tests. In fact, he didn't want to talk to me at all, and sat in the back of the ambulance not talking; at one point he threatened to leave the ambulance but I managed to persuade him otherwise. (Don't ask me why, I normally let drunks go as soon as they say they don't want to go to hospital.)

All went as normal until we rounded the corner to the hospital, where he got off of the chair and laid on the trolley-bed. One-hundred yards later and we pulled up to the hospital and I told him to get up, then I told him louder, then I did a sternal rub to wake him up—and there was no response! I

119

then slipped an oropharyngeal airway into his mouth, this would wake anyone up, but not a flicker . . . he was deeply unconscious. This meant he was due for the Resus' room.

We rolled him (rather quickly) into the Resus' room and were met by a rather angry nurse—she wanted to know why we hadn't pre-alerted the hospital, I explained that he had just lost consciousness outside the department. She then asked me why he didn't have oxygen on him. Again, I repeated that he had collapsed when we were outside the hospital. We got him onto one of their Resus' trolleys while the doctors in the department ran into the room.

For the third time I explained what had happened, and that I had no vital sign observations; this time they paid attention, and accepted what had happened.

To be honest I don't blame them, the A&E department rarely has any surprises—the hospital is normally forewarned about any 'nasty job' we are bringing them, and to suddenly have a seriously sick patient turn up without any warning is always a bit of a jolt.

Now the patient was unconscious the nurses were able to do those vital observations that I was unable to do—and they were all normal. His pulse, blood pressure and blood oxygen levels were all better than mine, his blood sugar was also well within normal limits. There was no obvious reason why he was in such a deep state of unconsciousness.

He was quickly intubated, and we left the department. I've spent some time wondering if I missed anything—if there was anything I would have done differently—but to be honest I don't think there was. Even if I had managed to get a full set of vital sign observations, they would have all been normal and there was nothing that indicated his condition changing so quickly. I can't 'assault' a patient who has refused a procedure (such as observation taking), and all I could do was exactly what I did do—watch him while we took him to hospital.

The current idea is that he had taken an overdose of some sort along with the alcohol, and that it had started to work. Because the patient hadn't spoken to me, I had no way of knowing if he had taken an overdose.

I never did find out what had happened with the patient—it's one of the poor things about this job, that you can't always follow them up.

PROTECTING LITTLE OLD MEN FROM THE POLICE?

We were asked go to the local police station to help with arresting someone. The arrestee (is that a real word?) was an 80 (or more)-year-old male who was accused of recently committing a crime that I would suggest required some amount of physical strength. We were to follow along because the person had heart and breathing problems—so much so that he had bottled oxygen in his house.

We met with the police officers (nine in total, and all rather scary looking plain-clothes types) at the police station, before following them to the address in question.

Once the police had made their entrance we

were called forward to give the patient a clean bill of health. We watched as this frail man slowly dressed, needing help from his son to tie his shoelaces; we watched as he struggled around the house and wondered how he could possibly be guilty of any crime that needed any form of physical exertion.

The patient's son was also a bit put out by the allegations, and promised to have a good laugh at the police's expense when the truth came out.

Throughout the arrest the police were polite, helpful and behaved in a thoroughly professional manner at all times.

The patient/arrestee was also calm throughout and the whole thing went, as far as I could see, very smoothly, and our ambulance followed the car in which he was taken, until it entered the police station and the FME (Forensic Medical Examiner—a doctor that the police use) took over.

The next job we went to was to outside the same address: a woman had been mugged and the police who were searching the address had called us as she had a rather large bump on her head. Unfortunately, the mugger managed to get away. It surprises me that you can get mugged outside a house full of police and the mugger can still escape.

VICTIMS

Imagine, if you will, getting sent to a job where a 15-year-old boy is threatening suicide. You turn up at the address and discover that it is a care home. Meeting with one of his carers she hands you a list of the boy's medications and it reads like a 'Who's

Who' of psychiatric drugs. You talk to the boy, and he seems calm, collected and very polite. He explains that he wants to jump out of a window and kill himself, and agrees that he would like to go to hospital. You take him into the paediatric department of a local hospital. As this does not feel like the normal 'Teenager wants to kill themselves' you have a chat with the children's nurse and you ask them to let you know what happens to the patient. You leave, and continue with your shift. The next day you ask the children's nurse about the patient and she tells you 'The boy wanted to die because he wants to have sex with, and kill small children—and that he knows that it is wrong'.

I hate paedophiles as much as any other member of society, but in front of me that day, I saw a victim.

🚑 BEHIND LOCKED DOORS

One of the jobs that I both enjoy and hate is for a 'Collapse behind locked doors'. This is when a (normally elderly) patient has not answered the front door or the telephone, and is presumed to be in some trouble. What we often get is someone who has died during the night. Although I hate having people die, the one good thing about this type of job is that I get to use my size 12 boots to kick down a door.

There is a skill to kicking down a door, and I was taught by the best—a policeman. The police also have a huge ram that they can use when their boots aren't enough. These are very heavy, but also lots of fun to use.

We got called to a house where the daughter could see her elderly mother lying on the floor; shouting through the door and banging on windows didn't get any response, so we assumed the worst. The daughter was (understandably) crying, so I had an attempt at kicking the door down.

Unfortunately for me, the woman had been burgled earlier in the year, and so had two locks, and a bolt holding the door shut, so it took a couple of minutes of prolonged (and eventually painful) kicking to get the door open. I also managed to wake up all the neighbours, and it's always fun to be the centre of attention . . .

Finally, the door gave and we gained access, we were greeted by the elderly woman sitting on the floor smiling at us—earlier in the morning she had fallen and couldn't get up. When we had tried banging on her windows she had been asleep, and it was only the repeated bashing of my foot against her door that had caused her to wake up.

This was a good job in a number of ways: the lady was happy and healthy, and just needed a hand to get up off of the floor; I got to kick in a door and get away with not causing any serious damage; and finally we looked like heroes to the two daughters of our patient. There were smiles all round and we left the job feeling that we had really been of some use today.

🚐 SUBSTITUTE

I know that the ambulance service is being used as a substitute GP service these days, but it really takes the biscuit sometimes. Take, for example, the job I was sent on last night. It came down to our ambulance as 'Patient wants to kill his doctor'.

I immediately called up Control on the radio and asked if we were being sent because they couldn't find the patient's GP? Although I was half joking, I wondered what good we could do for the patient. Control got back to us, and let us know that they were sending the police, and that we should wait until they turn up. However, when we arrived at the address we knew who the patient was—so we cancelled the police and sorted out the patient's problem.

I mention this if only because, when I got back on station and read the local newspaper, I found a story about a coroner's investigation into the death of a 55-year-old female who had taken a fatal overdose of bloodpressure medication. When Control asked if she was violent, they were told that yes, the patient was violent. The police were called and the crew waited at a rendezvous point for half an hour until the police turned up. By then it was too late, and the patient died. Once more, the paper blames the ambulance crew. It doesn't blame the psychiatric services who discharged her a few weeks earlier after a failed suicide attempt, neither does it blame the person who made the phone call that said that the patient was violent. It blames the crew who, quite rightly, waited for the police. If one of the crew had been stabbed to death, it might be a more sympathetic headline. We are expected to go into people's houses, where we have been told that the patient is violent, where we could get assaulted or even killed—but as soon as we start thinking about our own safety, *we* are the ones to blame for anything that goes wrong with that patient.

Violence from the drunks, druggies and criminals doesn't worry me—the job that worries me is the little old lady who has become confused and is sitting in her living room with her husband's service revolver, or her favourite kitchen knife, desperate to stop the strange men in green from stealing her away in the night.

As normal the ambulance service has investigated, but in a show of support for its road staff, has stated that the policy of waiting for the police at a rendezvous point is the correct thing to do.

We are not cowards, but neither are we stupid/paid enough to wander into dangerous situations.

☕ NICKED

I've just gotten on station for the start of my shift, only to find out that some scrote had broken into the station last night and nicked the video recorder and DVD player.

I mean, it's not like we are ever on station long enough to use them, but it's the principle . . .

These are the sort of people that we serve, these are the sort of people we are polite, professional and caring towards—and this is how we are repaid . . .

� MORE NICKED

It's getting so you have to tie things down now . . .
Yesterday a 'Decontamination POD' truck was

stolen; this is an unmarked truck that we use to carry around chemical incident equipment. The current word is that this truck was carrying a load of atropine, which is the treatment for nerve agents.

If people were to start injecting this into themselves, they could get serious (as in fatal) effects.

I leave it as an exercise for the reader to decide if this is a good or a bad thing . . .

YOU DECIDE

Still no drunks, but, the weekend starts today and my shift ends at 2 a.m . . .

I'm going to describe a job I went to last night.

The patient is female and 30 years old. She is married and is attempting to get pregnant. The only medicine she is taking is fertility treatment, and she is (obviously) having unprotected sex; she is normally fit and healthy and has no allergies. Her normal menstrual period is regular, but her period is over 2 weeks late this time around. She has been having nausea and vomiting for the past 3 days. She has no abdominal pain, and is not tender or guarding. She has no pain or increased frequency of passing urine. All vital signs are within normal limits.

So . . . given this information . . .

(a) What do you think is 'wrong' with her?

(b) Does she need a trip to hospital in an ambulance?

(c) Why do you think she hasn't done a pregnancy test?

🚑 DRAGGING

Sometimes a day can just drag along. Today, due to rather unusual circumstances, the day really dragged. Here is the time-line of today:

10:00 Turn up for work, brew a cup of tea.

10:01 First job of the day, taking someone from Newham hospital to St Barts hospital.

10:02 Cut my finger on my locker door, try to stop bleeding, look for plaster.

10:23 Give up search for a plaster—there are none on the station—leave for Newham hospital.

10:26 Arrive at Newham hospital, ask for plaster; they also don't have a plaster so I now have a huge dressing on my finger.

10:28 Meet with patient, pleasant woman—meet nurse who will be accompanying patient, barely understand nurse because of her inability to speak English.

10:30 Get patient's notes and read them—they make more sense.

10:32 Ask nurse in charge why this patient (who is having cardiac monitoring and a blood transfusion) is going to an outpatient department. Get told that the patient 'just is'.

10:54 After packaging the patient on a stretcher, loading them on the back of the ambulance, we set off for St Barts hospital.

10:55 Nurse escort tells me that she gets travel sick.

10:55 and 20 seconds Give nurse a vomit bag.

11:37 Arrive at St Barts hospital.

11:38 Enter outpatients' department, Reception seem rather surprised to see patient on stretcher appear in front of them.

11:40 Problem is referred to the sister in charge, she also looks befuddled.

12:00 We wait while sister in charge phones around the hospital trying to work out why this patient is in her outpatient department.

12:30 Still waiting . . . We let Control know why we are waiting—there is no stretcher/bed to put the patient on.

13:00 Still waiting.

13:30 Still waiting—we let Control know that we still have the patient on our stretcher while they work out what they are going to do with our patient.

14:00 Still waiting.

14:30 Still waiting—we let Control know that we haven't gone to sleep, we are told by sister in charge that patient will be admitted soon.

14:45 We place patient on an examination bed so that we can go back to answering emergency calls; patient will hopefully be in a hospital bed soon. We leave the nurse escort with the patient.

14:48 We are finally available for another job.

14:49 We realise we have nearly no fuel, and no fuel card to pay for fuel. We decide to return to station to borrow a fuel card off an unused ambulance.

15:20 We arrive back on station to look for fuel card (and have a cup of tea).

15:30 We leave to get fuel. Take infusion pump back to hospital—the ward seem surprised that the patient has been admitted to St Barts.

15:48 We have fuel, we are now ready for another job.

16:00 We get a call, out of area Matern-a-taxi.

16:09 Arrive at Matern-a-taxi, contractions

(genuinely) every 2 minutes, previous baby born in 3 *hours*, drive rather quickly toward her booked hospital.

16:12 Patient's waters break—start swimming in back of ambulance.

16:20 Arrive at hospital.

16:24 Throw patient at midwife, run back to ambulance.

16:30 Tell Control that we need to return to station to mop out the back of the ambulance.

17:20 Get back to station, mop out.

17:45 Crew to relieve us are already on station; await ambulance to dry out.

18:00 Leave for home.

18:37 Get home, collapse into sofa, start writing this post.

- Fin -

This is how you get to work an 8-hour shift, yet only do two jobs . . .

After this post I got given a box of plasters by a fellow blogger. No more searching around ambulance stations for sticking plasters.

SEDATION

I should be working today, but (and I want loads of sympathy here folks) I'm off sick with a work-related injury. Thankfully, it's nothing too serious, certainly nothing as serious as last time when I swallowed HIV-positive blood.

On Thursday we got called to a big conference centre in town for a (possibly) suspended/dead/fitting male. We rushed over there and were met by their security who had rather cleverly staked out both entrances to this place so that they could lead us to the patient. Parking up we had to climb a couple of flights of stairs carrying nearly all the equipment from the ambulance. Our first-response bag, oxygen and associated kit, defibrillator, suction and carry-chair are quite heavy and, as we were in a rush to get up the stairs, we were a bit out of breath when we reached the patient.

The first thing that we saw (and were *very* happy about) was that the patient had not suspended, and was instead thrashing around on the floor with some security guards and the centre's medic sitting on top of him. Approaching closer we saw that he wasn't fitting, but was instead very combative, trying to fight off the people who were holding him down in a very confused nature. Aha! we thought, 'he's post-ictal'.

During the post-ictal phase of a seizure, the fitting has stopped, but the patient is often disorientated, sleepy or aggressive. In this case it appeared that the patient was both confused and aggressive—he was not responding to anyone trying to talk to him to calm him down, and he could only make guttural sounds. Normally, these episodes last less than half an hour, so we stay with the patient until we can get them into the ambulance.

Sometimes the aggression can come from physically being held down—the patient is confused and frightened, and all they can feel is people holding them down, so they struggle. I suggested that the security guards let him go, which resulted in the patient trying to stand up, only to fall over again (don't worry, we caught him) and unfortunately the centre medic got a head butt for his trouble. I managed to get a blood glucose reading, which was normal, and a work colleague phoned the patient's mother, so I could get a bit of history. The patient is normally fit and healthy, not diagnosed with epilepsy, but has had two fits in the past 2 years. All during this phone conversation the mother could hear her son shouting in the background. He had never been violent before.

We resigned ourselves to a bit of a wait, so we managed to get him over to a leather couch, and held him down there. After 10 minutes there was no change in the patient's condition—normally they get a bit tired or they start to have a change in their condition. So we started to think about other ways in which we could help the patient at the scene. We couldn't get him to the ambulance while he was so combative, and so we thought he might need some form of sedation. I ran back to the ambulance and asked control to get us a BASICS doctor, or at least someone who could give some form of sedation.

Instead after about 10–15 minutes we got the PRU (Physician Response Unit), which is a new service where a doctor from the Royal London Hospital covers medical emergency calls—it's a bit like HEMS, only without the helicopter, and instead of going to trauma they mainly deal with medical emergencies.

The doctor (who is a very nice man) and paramedic crew with him took one look at the patient, listened to the history and decided that sedation was a very good idea.

Cut forward 40 minutes' worth of trying to sedate the patient with increasing amounts of medication. For the medically trained out there, the patient needed 10 mg haloperidol and 17 mg of midazolam. At one point the doctor was thinking about knocking the patient completely out and intubating him. Luckily the patient was sedated enough for us to get him out of the conference centre and into out ambulance, where we 'blued' him into Newham hospital just in time for him to wake up (the sedation lasting only around 15 minutes) where the doctors there did paralyse and intubate him.

We have few ideas why the patient was so violent and so deeply confused—its something that will be investigated in hospital. We were considering epilepsy, head trauma (from when his head hit the floor), meningitis (so antibiotics were given on scene) or some form of brain insult. I'm asking my crewmate to find out what happened to the patient.

The reason why I am off sick? Well after holding the patient down for an hour and 10 minutes, I managed to sprain my thumb. Since I can't be considered safe to carry a patient downstairs, I'm taking today off (plus 2 days of leave) so that my thumb can heal and I can get back to saving lives picking up drunks again on Monday. Oh, and it's my birthday tomorrow—33 is such a young age don't you think?

I did manage to see the patient again . . . see the next entry.

🚐 PATIENT GETS BETTER!!!

I went to visit our patient from the last post. This morning I'd put my hand in my pocket and found that I had £2.66 of his money that had spilled out of his pocket during our struggle and I'd put it in my fleece for safe keeping—given the saga of the job, I'd forgotten to hand it in when we reached the hospital. I thought it would be best if I returned it to him, so I had a chat with the lovely receptionists at the hospital, and they told me what ward he was on.

I went to the ward to find him sitting there, seemingly none the worse for wear. He did have a bit of a black eye (not my fault . . . honest), and when I spoke to him he told me that the doctors suspected that he had fainted, and when he had hit his head had suffered a form of concussion. His CT scan and blood tests were all normal, although I suspect that they will be running EEGs (electroencephalograms) and other more detailed tests a little later. He told me that he was feeling pretty much normal and I suspect that they are keeping him in hospital to continue to run their tests.

He was very pleased to see me, and we had a little chat. I offered him his money but he refused and suggested that I get myself a pint with it.

It's the first time I've actively gone to look for a patient after bringing them into hospital—and it is a weird experience going into a ward to see a patient whom I last saw trying to fight me. Yet another new thing I've done because of writing this blog.

🚑 SAFETY NET

I've mentioned before how the ambulance service and the A&E department are often seen as a 'safety net' by other health-care providers. Both yesterday and today we had perfect examples of this.

Yesterday we were called by a 70-year-old man with a urinary catheter which had blocked. This is a fairly simple thing to solve as it just needs a flush of water up the catheter to clear the blockage. It's a 5-minute job that we, as ambulance crews, aren't allowed to do. However it is the sort of job that district nurses are supposed to do.

So why hadn't a district nurse been to see the patient so that she could flush the catheter and prevent the patient from having to attend A&E? Why was the patient, who had phoned up the nurse himself, and told her exactly what he needed doing, forced to call an ambulance?

Because the nurse didn't have any water to actually flush the catheter. It's a bit like if I turned up to someone having an asthma attack, and didn't have any oxygen to give them.

So the district nurse told the patient to dial 999 for an ambulance. We arrived and found him with a bladder so full it was causing him severe pain. We took him into Newham hospital, who, within minutes had cleared his catheter, and eased his pain. They gave him a 'takeaway' bottle of water so that the district nurse wouldn't have an excuse the next time she needed to visit him.

Today, we were called to a patient who needed his anti-Parkinson's disease medication. He had a carer, who was supposed to visit him once a day to clean, and arrange his medication. But for the last 2 days, because the 'carer' couldn't get in touch with the patient's GP, she'd just left him without his medication. We turned up, not knowing what

135

we could do to help. The flat in which the patient was living is brand new, and yet was already very untidy. The patient told me that he was lucky if the carer spent longer than 5 minutes with him (the carer is contracted to work with him for an hour a day).

This poor man was left, alone and shaking, with a carer who seemed to think that if she ignored this 'problem' it would soon go away. So, we did the only thing that we could: we took him to hospital, so that they could sort out his medication for him. Meanwhile I filled in an 'LA260' which is a 'vulnerable adults' form and allows the LAS to bring situations of abuse, and potential abuse, to the attention of the local social services. They now have the name of the care agency, and this problem can be solved before it repeats itself in a month's time.

Hopefully, someone will get a bollocking, and our patient will get a carer who actually cares for him.

It often feels that we, and the local A&E departments, are left to do the jobs that other people should be doing, but because we are there, these other agencies don't seem to care about doing a competent job. I'm aware that there are probably loads of health visitors/social workers/district nurse/CPNs and GPs who do actually give a damn about their patients—it's just that we never seem to meet them.

I never did get any feedback from the LA260 that I filled in—normally you get a little note sent to you explaining what has been done to resolve the situation.

🚐 A HIDDEN PREGNANCY

Our 'interesting' call of last night was a Matern-a-taxi. What, I hear you ask could be interesting about taking a pregnant woman 1.2 miles into the local maternity department?

Well, apart from the patient, no-one else knew that she was pregnant—she had been hiding the pregnancy from everyone. She hadn't seen a doctor; neither had she booked into a maternity department. Her family suspected nothing. It's not as if she were a 'large' woman, who could perhaps hide the tell-tale bump under the pretence of fat. She was actually rather slender, which leads me to ask how she could hide her rather obvious pregnancy from everyone.

When my crewmate spoke to her (I was driving), she told him that she had hoped that the pregnancy would 'go away'.

We tried to prewarn the maternity department that we were coming (because she was quite close to actually delivering the baby), but they hung up the phone twice on our Control. The problem is that the entrance to the maternity department is locked at night, and we need someone to come down and open it for us. So . . . we were left standing around outside the department waiting for the midwives to phone for a porter to traipse the length of the hospital to come and open the door for us (as opposed to one of the midwives walking down the stairs and opening the door).

By the time we got in the patient was starting to bleed, and we were getting more irate at the apparent ignorance of the midwives.

So, tonight we are going to put in a 'clinical

incident report' to highlight the danger that standing outside the maternity department for 10 minutes while they arrange a porter puts the patient in.

One of the people on Complex has had to deliver a baby in the back of their ambulance while they were waiting for the doors to be opened, so something needs to be done.

🚐 UPSETTING

Three of our jobs today had the potential to be upsetting, and while they were all sad, only one seriously upset me, and did so in a way I consider rather out of character for myself.

The first job of the day was to an 86-year-old female in a nursing home with a 'blocked nose': we raced around there because . . . well . . . it was a Category 'A' call and those are the top-priority 'get there in 8 minutes to please the government target' calls.

Just as we pulled up outside Control let us know that the patient was upgraded to a 'Suspended' (no pulse, no breathing), and sure enough we ran into the home to be greeting by a FRU who was doing CPR. I jumped down and did a round of chest compressions, which cracked her ribs (a recognised side-effect of effective CPR) and then noticed that on the cardiac monitoring machine her heart rhythm had changed. She had a pulse! . . . People don't normally get a pulse back from cardiac arrests of her particular type. We rushed her to the hospital, where a full cardiac arrest team was assembled. Her pulse was lost, and then returned.

Unfortunately, her prognosis was poor, but she stayed alive long enough for her daughter to reach the hospital. She died with her daughter there, which is a small victory, but one that we are getting more used to. The second potentially upsetting job was to a 1-year-old boy who had pulled some boiling milk on top of him. We turned up to find about 20 police officers on scene, and the HEMS helicopter circling above. The same FRU responder was there and the child had around 10% partial thickness burns to parts of the neck and chest. While nasty, this wasn't immediately life-threatening, but the HEMS doctor who turned up decided that it would be best to take the patient to the Paediatric Burns Unit at Chelsea and Westminster Hospital by helicopter. As the helicopter could get the child there in under 20 minutes it seemed like the right plan of action. My job during this call was to (1) hold onto the other two toddlers in the house, (2) mix up some paracetamol for the child, and (3) drive child and doctor to the helicopter, which was around 300 yards away. The job was interesting because she was the type of parent who thought it was a good idea to wedge a settee into the hallway to stop her children from falling down the stairs . . .

The final job was a lot simpler—we were called to an 18- to 22-year-old female who was 'unresponsive' in a bus. The bus had reached the end of its route and the driver couldn't wake up the patient. (Possibly interesting aside—bus drivers cannot touch any of their customers to wake them up.) We turned up and soon managed to wake up the very sleepy girl. She remained drowsy but agreed to let us take her to the place where she lived, but after talking to her a bit, we soon realised that she was homeless. This, coupled with the way she would fall asleep as soon as we stopped talking to her, made us think that it would not be safe to leave her on the street. We decided instead that we would take her to hospital. When we reached the hospital she refused to go in, and instead pulled out a 'crack' pipe and started to light up. We told her that she couldn't do that . . . So she jumped up, pushed my crewmate and ran off. As there was nothing physically wrong with her we couldn't chase after her; instead we returned to our station to fill in the necessary paperwork.

So why was it that this last job was the most upsetting, not only for myself but also for my crewmate? Well it wasn't because she was pretty (she wasn't, and she had a remarkably nasal voice), and it wasn't because she was ill, neither was it because my crewmate got shoved.

With our first job, the woman was at the end of her life, and until she died, had enjoyed fairly good health. She didn't die a painful, protracted death, and she died with her daughter next to her. With the scalded child, he would forget the pain, and will receive excellent care from the hospital he went to, he would return home to his loving (if ever so slightly dense) mother. With this girl, it was as if she were lost; at some point in her life her potential future had unravelled. Instead of getting an education, holding down a job, finding someone special and living a long and happy life, she is homeless, a drug addict, and her future is probably painful and short. What is so depressing is that no-one was able to turn around this descent, and this is perhaps why I despair at society—that so many

140

people are prevented from reaching their full potential. I understand that she has made her own choices, but how much power did she have to make those choices? I wanted to help her, but there was no way I could do this.

And it's that which annoyed and upset me.

I keep getting upset and annoyed at the same things—the waste of a life is a terrible thing to see. That, and the knowledge that I am helpless to do anything to change it. I imagine that this is why I dislike alcoholics so much.

🚐 THERAPY?

We got sent to a job of a 6-month-old baby not breathing. While this often means that baby has a cold, it could also be one of the worse jobs you can get. We sped to the address and entered a house where the whole family was distraught. It was an Indian household, so there were a lot of people there, and most of them were crying. Once more, I heard the type of crying that can only mean that something awful has happened—entering the living room I instantly saw a baby lying dead on the settee, father crouched over it crying and the mother standing and wailing, shouting out that her baby was dead.

There is only one thing that you can do in a situation like this, which is to scoop up the baby and run to hospital as quickly as possible. I reached down and picked up the baby; I was shocked to find that it was as stiff as a board and very purple, indicating that it had been dead for some time. It looked more like a doll than anything that had once been alive. We could have recognised the child as dead on the scene, but taking the child to hospital would mean that the parents would see that everything that could be done was being done and, more importantly, they would be in a hospital with all the support that the hospital could provide.

I ran out to the ambulance with mother in tow, and told my crewmate to get us to hospital as quickly as possible. The father and grandmother followed behind us in another ambulance who had heard this call go out and had turned up to see if there was anything that they could do to help. On the way to hospital I did the CPR that I knew was ultimately pointless and spoke to the mother. She had last seen the child alive at 3 a.m., and he had been fine then. It looked like it may have been a case of sudden infant death syndrome, and I did all that I could to prepare the mother for the worst.

We pulled up at hospital and handed the baby into the care of the hospital. I spoke a little more with the mother and grandmother, but there is nothing that you can say to people who have had such a tragedy. Our station officer met us at the hospital and asked us if we were alright, then he booked us off the road so that we could go back to station and have a cup of tea and 'decompress'. If we needed more support I think it would have been there, but I just wanted to get away from the hospital.

I'm not often affected by jobs, and this isn't the first dead baby that I've had to deal with, but it is the first dead baby I've had since joining the ambulance service and it is very different from dealing with them in hospital. Going into someone's house to take away a dead child is very different from having the child and parents turn up at hospital, which is your safe territory.

At the hospital all the other crews were asking if I was alright and, to be honest, I wasn't really alright—I was upset that while I was doing CPR on the baby its legs were seesawing into the air, and it looked too much like a doll. There was a point after the job where I thought I was going to start crying, but a moment outside the Resus' room and I was back to functioning as I normally do. I'm not weak, and when in the midst of something I can deal with anything—it was only after the doctors and nurses at the hospital had taken over that I started to feel anything.

We returned to station, where the therapy of talking about anal surgery with another crew, and a cup of tea soon had me feeling better. It used to be that you would return to work straight after a job like this, but then I think they realised that if we got our normal inappropriate call (belly-ache for 2 weeks sort of thing) we might say something to the patient that we might later regret.

Well, an hour on station later and I feel fully prepared to deal with that sort of thing again—but I think that I'll be haunted by the image of that child lying dead on my trolley.

I had loads of people commenting on this post, loads of support, which was very much appreciated. The title is a reference to the fact that I have found my blog to be 'therapy' for some of the things that I've seen and done in the ambulance service . . . and it's cheaper than hitting the bottle.

I've often mentioned that the ambulance service and the police tend to get on rather well together, this is at least in part due to us both being called to the same jobs, and probably because we share the same view of the 'Great British Public'.

An example: we got called to a drunk who was being verbally abusive to a bus driver—we were called because the drunk had fallen over, while the police were called because of the abuse. The drunk man was obnoxious, and well known to both of our services, and because of the lack of an injury was left in the care of the police. If he had been injured then the police would have left the matter in our hands.

So, when we co-respond, the ambulance crew pray that the patient is uninjured, so the police have to deal with them, while I suspect that the police hope that the patient is injured so they don't have to arrest them.

However, there are a lot of specialist teams in the police service that we tend not to come into contact with that often; we mainly get to meet the normal 'beat' coppers. Thankfully, we rarely see the murder, child abuse, drugs or dog teams. This isn't to say we never see them (and our station did get a Christmas card from the local murder squad telling us to 'keep up the good work'), it's just that it is fairly rare.

So, it was rather surprising that I met with the dog-handling team twice last week. On the first occasion, we were called to a known schizophrenic who had threatened to kill herself. The patient herself (a regular attender at the local A&E) was a bit of a pain to deal with, she wanted to stay at home and kill herself and couldn't see why we wouldn't let her do that. Her dog, on the other hand, was a real pleasure—happy to see us, interested in smelling all our equipment and extremely friendly. As the police were already there, they got the dog squad to look after the animal until the patient was discharged from hospital.

In case you think I am being harsh on the mentally ill, the patient attends A&E every day with the same complaint of wanting to kill themselves . . . she hasn't managed it yet.

The second time I saw the dog-handling team was when we had to gain access to a house where the patient was unable to come to the front door and let us in. The interesting part in this story is that there were five dogs of unknown temperament in the house. For half an hour the police unsuccessfully tried to gain access, mainly by climbing up a ladder and trying to open a bathroom window. We were able to talk to the patient, and so we knew that they were not badly hurt, otherwise we would have had to kick the door down. Then the dog team turned up and, using a top secret criminal technique, managed to get the front door open in about 10 seconds, thus putting to shame the half-hour everyone else had spent trying to gain entry.

All five dogs were really lovely, although energetic, and at the end of the job I had to spend 20 minutes brushing the dog hair off my uniform.

There is a joke we have about dogs. When we ask a patient if the dog is friendly, the patient *always* answers that they won't bite, the reply to this from the ambulance crew is to add the unspoken 'They only bite people dressed all in green'.

I've only had one dog take a dislike to me. But I managed to pull my hands away from his gnashing teeth before he could catch me.

PERILS OF DRINKING (NUMBER 1 IN A SERIES OF 230)

It was the usual type of busy last night—we heard rumours that there is such a thing as an 'ambulance station', a mythical building where one might use the toilet or partake of the life-giving 'cup of tea'. It must be a myth, as we never saw it at all.

As I have mentioned, we get our calls sent down to a computer screen in the ambulance cab; sometimes you wonder how the Control crew have entered it while keeping from laughing down the phone at the patient. A case in point was one of our calls last night which was given as '53-year-old male, taken 3 x crack cocaine, cold and lonely, needs to be put back together'.

Avoiding the rather obvious 'Humpty Dumpty' jokes, we soon realised that the complaint, and the location he was calling from, fitted one of our semiregular callers. By the time we got there he had left the phone box and neither us nor the police could find him after a search of the area. Obviously I was distraught . . .

Our other stand-out job of the night was a 57-year-old male fitting. We quickly made our way to the location, to be met by a block of low-rise flats that often sneak up on you in our area. These are three or four floors high, and have no lifts. Also there was one of our First Responders. We entered the block, and immediately made our way to the stairs (it is a little known law of physics that in flats with no lifts, people on the ground floor are never ill . . . only those on the top floor).

Entering the flat, the general state of disrepair, mess and the 3-litre bottle of strong cider I tripped over tended to give the impression that it was owned by an alcoholic. We got into the living room to find a large man lying senseless on the floor, while his daughter was sat over him stroking his hand, trying to reassure him. A quick check over, some oxygen and a chat with his daughter revealed a history of alcoholism (surprise!) and the occasional alcoholic fit. He was a big man, so we packaged him up in our carry-chair and carried him down three flights of stairs. All the time his daughter was saying how strong the nice ambulance men were—which only goes to show that she wasn't paying attention to my reddening face and struggles for breath . . .

We got the patient into the back of the ambulance where he started to fit again, this time lasting about 2 minutes. He also decided to bite his tongue and vomit, which meant that the back of the ambulance (and myself in some part) was covered in bloody, cider-smelling vomit. I think I've mentioned before how I can't smell alcohol on someone's breath, yet I can smell cider when it has been vomited all over my ambulance . . . and it turns my stomach. We packaged him up and 'blued' him into Newham, where he had another two fits (despite some rather strong sedation) and by the end of our shift he was still in Resus' having

147

infusions of phenytoin and Pabrinex.

So, a busy night without the chance to see our station, with at least one mopping out of the ambulance . . . pretty standard really.

The vomit in the ambulance took place at the end of our shift, so we couldn't even get back to station to use the mop. Unfortunately, with the increased number of calls we have, getting back to station is becoming rarer than ever.

SECURITY

Yes, I know I've written before about kicking down doors. However, in this post I offer people advice in making the beating down of their door as hard as possible. So please excuse the repetition. Like all good health-care professionals I regularly ignore my own advice.

There is a visceral pleasure in kicking down a door. Once or twice I've managed to see someone who is really ill trapped behind a locked door, occasionally there has been someone who has just been unable to open the door. And just the once I have kicked down a door that the patient refused to open because they were schizophrenic and didn't want to open the door—not that I knew that at the time.

I've even been surprised at the ease in which I can kick down the doors of the flats that I live in. Actually, it would be more accurate to say that I am *scared* with the ease in which the doors can be broken. Oh well, it's not as if I have a lot to steal anyway . . .

My experience of kicking down doors has taught

me which security features are useful when trying to prevent someone from stealing your TV and video.

If you have a deadlock-type lock, then use it— always. The skill of kicking down a door relies on breaking either the lock, or the wood holding the lock; deadbolt-type locks are a lot more secure than the normal Yale type lock.

If you are in the house and have a bolt on the door, then use it. It takes a lot longer to kick down a door when there is a bolt in the way. Another trick behind kicking down a door relies on applying the force of your kick to the (hopefully) single point of resistance. If there is a bolt at the top, or the bottom of the door it makes it a lot trickier to break that door.

Windows in the door are a bad idea—they are a weak point that can be easily broken, and then a skinny hand can reach through and unlock the door.

If you really want to be safe then have a bar across the door. I've seen it once or twice, and if someone had a bar across the door then there is no way I'd be able to break that door down. Just make sure you don't collapse behind it.

🚐 MAJOR INCIDENT COVER

One of the perks of this job is the need to cover football games. Well . . . it's a perk if you enjoy seeing your local team play. Personally, I can't stand football but overtime is overtime, and it does make a nice change from the usual jobs I go to. So, this Sunday I got to see West Ham play against Derby.

The LAS provide 'Major Incident' cover for these games, we don't look at sprained ankles or minor injuries (that is the job of the St John's ambulance). We also don't look after the players who get hacked down and are unable to walk, only to watch them turning somersaults a scant 5 minutes later when their team scores a goal (that is a job for the private medical firms).

So, unless a stand collapses, there is a major fire, a bomb goes off or someone drops dead in front of us, there is very little we have to do. At the West Ham ground (my local football club), there are four 'road crew' present, along with at least one major incident support vehicle, one radio operator and an officer. The road crew sit down near the pitch, while the officer and radio operator sit in a VIP box overlooking the whole ground.

Today I was given the role of 'safety officer', which doesn't mean I've been promoted, it just means that in the event of a major incident, I'm supposed to watch out for the safety of the ambulance crews present, liaise with the police and fire service about any hazards that might be a problem, and to make sure that any crews that attend the incident are not getting too stressed. I also have to talk to the person in overall control at the incident about any issues within this sphere that may occur.

We were warned that there was an increased chance of violence at this match because some hooligan 'supporters' were appearing before the magistrate tomorrow, and that some of their 'crew' might want to cause some trouble. Luckily for us, that did not happen, despite a 2–1 loss.

It was really cold down there in the stands, I had

my undershirt, shirt, body armour, fleece and Hi-visibility all-weather jacket on, but I was still freezing. Anyone listening carefully as I walked around trying to keep warm would have heard a clink-clink-clink-clink sound as my frozen balls knocked together.

As I've mentioned before, I'm not a huge fan of football (overpaid idiots, getting more money in a week than I get paid in a year for booting around a plastic ball), so I spent most of the match listening to music (The Magnetic Fields) on my smart-phone, while stamping around trying to get some sensation back in my toes.

As a quick aside, who needs an iPod Shuffle? My smart-phone can do the same thing and more—it can even make phone calls . . .

Half-time came and went so we joined the St John's Ambulance for a cup of tea and a sandwich, rather than watch a bunch of scantily clad young women prance about. Then we were back in the cold, where I tried to stay awake while West Ham, perhaps predictably, lost . . .

With the exception of someone having a crafty cigarette and setting off a fire alarm, it all went rather smoothly. I did find it funny that the people in the stadium knew what the 'Inspector Sands' announcement meant, and did nothing but laugh quietly at it.

At the end of the match we have to stay around until we are 'stood down' as the last few supporters leave, so we sat in the ambulance, with the heater going, wrapped in our own blankets (remember, we know what those blankets have been wrapped around, yet we still used them—that is how cold it was).

151

We then started making our way back to station
. . .

. . . to come across a policeman who had tried to stop a car—only to have them speed up (possibly accidentally) and hit him. He wasn't especially badly hurt, but we took all precautions as we transported him to hospital. He'll need a few X-rays, but I suspect that he will be fine.

'Inspector Sands' is a codeword for use over a public address system. It is used to let the staff know that a fire alarm has gone off without alerting the public and possibly panicking them.

PHONETIC

I'm aware that because I am my own self-publicist I may come across as trying to sound 'perfect'. I will however blog about my mistakes . . . or at least the mistakes that won't lose me my job . . .

Part of our job involves using a radio to talk to Control, so part of our training is in the use of the radio. The training is about 3 hours long, and you spend it pretending to talk on a radio passing jobs back and forth (this is before the computer terminals were introduced).

One of the things we are taught is the phonetic alphabet, which I am sure you have all seen in film and TV. Normally, it sounds something like 'Foxtrot Alpha Sierra Tango Charlie Alpha Romeo', and is designed to make the spelling out of words over an unreliable radio transmission clearer and less likely to have errors.

One other thing that you should be aware of, is that our radio has an open broadcast: this means that everyone in the sector can hear you talking on it. You can recognise your friend's voices, and this radio chatter gives you a general idea of what they are doing. Of course, this means that should you make a mistake, everyone knows about it.

Why was it, when spelling out a name I suddenly forgot the phonetic for 'M' (Mike), and instead, in a moment of panic, decided that the new phonetic for 'M' would be . . .

. . . Mango?

It's not as if I have mangoes on the mind—I can't remember the last time I ate one—but for some reason it was the first thing that came into my mind.

I bless the radio operator for not bursting into laughter and calling me a twit.

ODDS AND ENDS

Today was typical, in that the jobs we did veered from interesting to dull, and from heartwarming to heartbreaking.

As an example of how one job can be different from another, we found ourselves attending an elderly man who was looked after by his daughter and son-in-law. They lived in Portugal, but when he had became ill they had moved back to England to look after him. The house was spotlessly clean, as was our patient; there was real love in the house and they obviously cared deeply for him. He was generally a bit poorly after a fall earlier in the day, so we took him to hospital for a check-up. Straight after that job, we ended up going to a pair of alcoholics living in squalor, where one of the pair had fallen over while drunk and had cut their ear. The patient later said that his partner had punched him, and that is why he had a cut ear, that and she had also kicked him in the stomach.

This is the fun bit of this job, we go from loving families to quarrelling drunken couples.

We had a bit of a 'trauma' with a victim of a hit-and-run. The patient was crossing the road when he got hit by a car, bounced up onto the bonnet and ended up in the middle of the road. Luckily, he wasn't hurt in a life-threatening way, but he did have a broken arm (for the medics in the audience, or those who can use Google, the patient had a simple transverse fracture of the mid-shaft humerus). He didn't have any other injuries, which in my book makes him rather lucky, especially considering the speed that cars can get up to down that particular road.

What was particularly interesting was that, although the man was lying in the middle of the very busy road, only a bus and one bystander had stopped—the bystander was making sure that he didn't get hit by any other cars. People were so unbothered that at one point I had buses rushing past my head as I treated him. You'd think people might slow their driving a little when swerving around an ambulance parked in the middle of the road with all its lights flashing . . .

But not around here they don't.

We also went to a 'Fire job', where a mother had left a 7-year-old, a 5-year-old and a 2-year-old locked alone in a house while she popped out for some fruit. A small fire had started, and the children had only been saved when a neighbour walked past and saw the kids crying at the window, and the orange flicker of flames in the background. He broke the window and saved the children. The mother was, perhaps unsurprisingly, distraught. A moment of carelessness nearly cost her children their lives. The quick thinking of the neighbour had meant that the children were completely unharmed, so I hope he gets a nice write-up in the local papers.

The final job of the day was to a 'nursing' home. The patient had apparently developed a bony lump under her hip. The staff thought that she might have broken her hip, but as the patient is bed-bound and as no-one admitted dropping her it would be a very suspicious fracture. I had a look at the supposed 'fracture' and couldn't see anything unusual, the patient was just extremely frail. The patient was suffering from dementia, and when I further examined her was also rather dehydrated. So we took her into hospital—along with a 'carer' from the home. All throughout the transport the patient was scared, so I did my best to look after her, hold her hand, talk to her, that sort of thing. During the journey the 'carer' stared out the window of the ambulance and didn't say a word apart from worrying that she would have trouble being relieved when her shift was finished.

When we left the patient at the hospital I told the 'carer' (can you see why I put 'carer' in quotes?) that her job now was to 'hold her hand, talk to her and reassure her because she would be scared in this unusual place. In fact, it gives you a chance to do that *caring* thing that you don't have time to do normally'.

I think she knew I was a bit angry at her but she did as I said, so maybe she got the point.

Another 12-hour shift tomorrow—then (hopefully) I'll have a day or two off, when I can sleep and perhaps manage to fix my laptop.

If the above post doesn't make any sense then tough, I'm knackered and all the Red Bull in the world can't make me into a Hemingway.

The man who saved the children did indeed get mentioned in glowing terms in the local paper. Once more I mention a lack of sleep and computer troubles, which along with a constant search for a nice cup of tea are the two constants in my life.

A CHANGED ROLE (THE SECRET IS OUT)

So, after some time (arranging things with work, battering my computer into submission and having a day of doing nothing except 'chilling out') I think I can finally reveal the 'big secret' that I have been using to keep you coming back to read this blog . . .

I'm still in the London Ambulance Service, and I've not been promoted; however, the vehicle that I drive, and the role that I play will change.

I'm no longer going to be driving one of these . . .

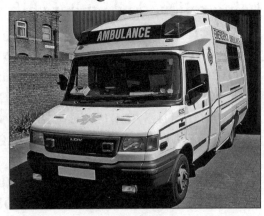

Or even one of these . . .

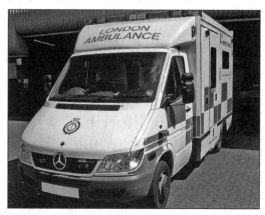

But one of these . . .

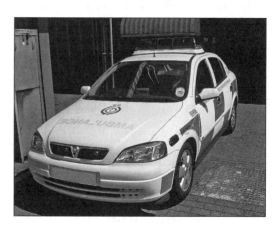

For the foreseeable future I am going to be on the Fast Response Unit (FRU).

The role of the FRU is to get to emergency calls within 8 minutes, thereby pleasing the government, and by extension, pleasing management.

I am to get to calls as quickly as possible, get a history off a patient and start treatment until an ambulance can arrive, then leave the patient in the care of the ambulance crew and drive off looking for another emergency call. When I don't have a call to go on, I am to spend at least some time driving around the area in the hope that I will be closer than an ambulance when a call does come in.

This means that I have even more autonomy than working on an ambulance, because I am working on my own—there is no crewmate to bounce ideas off. There is also a better chance of things going horribly wrong—imagine having to deal with a cardiac arrest on your own, with distraught relatives knowing that there isn't going to be an ambulance for 30 minutes . . .

Still . . . it should be fun, especially considering that I'm starting this new rota with a Friday, Saturday and Sunday night.

I stuck it for nearly a year before returning to an ambulance. Too much time spent on your own is bad for your mental health methinks. From here on in the posts are all about being an FRU pilot.

🚑 FIRST NIGHT

My first shift on 'the car' went fairly well. There are lots of things that are different between working from the car and working on a truck that I think you may be interested reading about, which means I'll have a series of postings about FRU work to write about when I next get some days off.

While others were dealing with stabbings and shootings (at least two in the area last night) I, who am supposed to go to the most serious calls, had two patients who actually needed hospital treatment, a crying baby, and five cases of 'D&V' (diarrhoea and vomiting). I was not alone in dealing with this sudden increase of D&V, Newham hospital was very busy with an epidemic of similar illness, and it seemed that crews were persuading a lot of them to stay at home and nurse themselves . . .

If you live in the area I work then I'd stay away from the kebab shops in Romford road (Manor Park end) if I were you, as at least 12 cases were tied to one kebab shop, with perhaps as many as 27 people eventually falling ill with the same symptoms after eating from the same shop.

Now . . . can I name the shop involved? Legally and ethically, am I on firm ground?

Maybe I should study journalism at night school . . .

I may have something more interesting tomorrow, but for the first night it was really pleasant to be eased into this entirely new way of working.

Now to sleep . . .

MAJOR FOOD POISONING INCIDENT —D&V PART 2

It turns out that Newham General Hospital had at least 70 people through their doors with the food poisoning epidemic. Some patients also had gone to King George's hospital or to Whipps Cross hospital, which, if you add in the number of people who are suffering in silence at home makes a lot of rather sick people.

The kebab place has duly been closed and the various public/environmental health bodies are looking closely at the situation. I have heard an unconfirmed rumour that the cause of the sickness was *Salmonella*.

159

At least one person is very ill, and at least eight people were admitted to Newham hospital. This has stretched the resources in the area to near breaking point, Newham hospital and King George's hospital were both closed on Sunday night because the A&Es were full, and there were no beds left in the hospital. It got so bad that Newham hospital declared an internal 'major incident'—a wise choice I think, as it means that the resources needed to deal with the situation are pointed in the right direction.

Unfortunately, with our local hospitals closed, patients have needed to go further to get to a hospital. Some are quite happy, such as those who get taken to the Royal London (in most people's eyes the Royal London is *the* hospital to go to). Meanwhile others have been less happy (such as those who have been taken to Whipps Cross).

It is my belief that a terrorist network doesn't need bombs to bring London to its knees, it just needs to spread a little *Salmonella* around, and then watch the NHS collapse.

It was a month or so later that the national news caught up on the story. Apparently the meat was contaminated at source and the kebab shop was blameless. Just one more example of how bloggers can move more quickly than more traditional media.

SHOPPING

I went out today and saw an alcoholic, a COPD (chronic obstructive pulmonary disease), a couple of heart failures, a handful of kids with chest infections and at least three anosmias (anosmia is a lack of a sense of smell).

The anosmia patients are those teenage girls who think that the best way to attract a slack-jawed mate is to empty half a bottle of cheap perfume over their heads—do they not know what they smell like?

However, I wasn't in an ambulance, and I wasn't on the FRU—in fact I wasn't working at all.

The answer is fairly simple—I just went shopping.

The problem with being surrounded by patients for 12 hours a day (first as a nurse, then to a lesser extent as an EMT), is that your eye is automatically drawn toward people with obvious symptoms. It's not just your eye—a trained ear can hear the cough of a child with a chest infection, or the puff and wheeze of a chronic bronchitis.

I suspect doctors have the same problem, the constant inspection of clubbing in the fingers, the subliminal inspection of the eyes and the unconscious appraisal of someone's gait.

In some part, it's because you are trained to look for what is wrong with people—but equally, there is that desire not to be around the person who is most likely to have a heart attack in front of you. At least when you are not on duty. This is why, when the 80-year-old female with ankles the size of tree trunks and blue lips decides to hit the pavement, there won't be a medical professional to be seen for miles.

It's not that we are lazy, or that we have no love for our fellow man when we are not getting paid for it, its just that without any of our 'kit', there is very little we can do to look busy, or effective. Without equipment, the options are CPR (if their heart has stopped), the recovery position (if they

161

are unconscious) or a 'there, there', with a bit of hand holding if it is a grazed knee.

Of course, the first thing to do is to call for an ambulance.

MOBILE PHONES

We often have problems with mobile phones in the ambulance service—we find ourselves trying to talk to a patient, while they are more intent on talking to their friend/mum/cousin/dealer on the phone.

I've had to pull people out of the way of incoming traffic because they are so focused on photographing the damage to their car with their mobile phone that they neglect to realise that they are standing in the middle of a busy dual carriageway.

I've been trying to resuscitate dead patients when their mobile phone has rung—I look at the screen and see that the person trying to call them is 'MUM'.

I've been in the middle of what can best be described as a 'public order situation', and while trying to deal with the injured (and prevent any more injuries), half the crowd are on the phone telling their 'posse' to get to that location as quickly as they can.

I've even had a patient and a relative fist-fighting in the back of my ambulance over an overheard phone call, made while the patient was pretending to be unconscious.

🚐 STANDBY

As the LAS doesn't have an ambulance station on every street, and given the state of London's roads and traffic, we find ourselves going out on 'Standby'.

Essentially ambulance crews and FRU cars are told to drive away from the station (with its heating, toilets and tea-making facilities) and sit in public roads to help cover a wider area. The idea is that because the 'resources' are spread out over a wider area you will be able to get to calls quicker, thus improving our all-important response time.

Crews don't like going out on standby, but I doubt anyone would like sitting in an ambulance cab waiting for someone to be ill/injured/drunk. Management like to have crews put out on standby because it apparently improves response times; this in turn pleases the government. I am yet to see some proper scientific evidence to back up this claim.

The standby points are chosen to be reasonably far away from station, around three miles in my case, and in an area where there is a reasonable expectation for there to be a high number of calls.

They also try to place you where a number of major road routes meet, so you can rapidly make your way out of your area to cover the shortfall in other sectors . . .

There are limits to how standby can be used. You can only be put on standby for 20 minutes at a time, and you can only be put on standby between the hours of 8 a.m. and 8 p.m., so while it is unpleasant to be put on standby, it isn't the complete torture that it could be.

On the FRU there is another ruling—that they can't spend longer than 30 minutes on station, so although I had five jobs over the space of 12 hours yesterday, I spent very little time actually on station. Most of my time was spent sitting behind Stratford shopping centre with the engine running so that I didn't freeze to death. When I got bored with that, I would roam the area, essentially looking for some trouble.

It is a fair assumption that it takes half an hour to do one job, from activation to being ready for the next job, so I was only actually working for two and a half hours since for an hour and a half I was on station, leaving me sitting in the car for 8 hours.

As I neared the end of my time on the FRU, one of my main problems was that I was getting severe back pain from sitting in a car for long periods of time. Management also wanted to change the times they could send the FRU on standby to 24 hours a day. Too dangerous for my liking.

WORTHWHILE (FOR A CHANGE)

Yesterday I felt that my role as a FRU was justified and this, coupled with the better weather, means that I am in a much better mood.

The unfortunate thing is that it was a tragedy that made me feel better.

The first job of the day came 2 hours into my shift, the call was 'Woman fell out of bed, not breathing'. I got to the house in 2 minutes and climbed the narrow stairs to find a 55-year-old woman lying in the lap of her daughter; also on the bed were two small children (perhaps 1 and 2 years

164

old). The younger woman was crying and my patient wasn't breathing.

I had to pull her out from the side of the bed so I could get my resuscitation attempt started—not very dignified, and probably not that nice to watch either, as a stranger in green pulls your mother across the floor.

I connected her to my heart monitor/ defibrillator, and saw that she was in PEA (pulseless electrical activity—a heart rhythm that means your heart isn't moving blood around your body and which is ultimately fatal), so I started chest compressions, and ventilating her with my Ambu-bag.

While doing this I was trying to get some form of medical history: none of her relatives could speak English that well, but I managed to gather that she had just rolled out of bed, and besides tablet-controlled diabetes she was otherwise healthy.

I was just about to finish the first round of CPR when I heard the ambulance crew turn up—I shouted down the stairs that the call was indeed a 'Suspended', and when they entered the room they started to intubate and try to gain venous access. Venous access means that we can give potentially life-saving drugs, but in this case the woman's veins were so small that after two attempts we realised that it wouldn't be possible. Instead, we were able to give her the drugs via the ET tube, which is the breathing tube we use to protect the patient's airway.

We then saw a change in her cardiac rhythm: from PEA she entered VF so we 'shocked' her with my defibrillator. She then went from PEA to VF and back again every time we shocked her.

165

At one point during transport to the hospital we got a pulse back, but this soon degenerated into VF.

The hospital worked on her for an hour, and at one point she had both a pulse and a blood pressure, but unfortunately she later died.

The memory of the job that I have is of cleaning her hair from where it had gotten stuck to the Ambu-bag, just after she had died in the hospital, hoping that the son-in-law wouldn't then choose that moment to look in the back of the ambulance.

At least I felt justified in my role. All too often you get used to being called to jobs that are, frankly, crap. This was a 'proper' job, and although we didn't save her, we gave her the best chance we could. If we hadn't been there then she wouldn't have had even that chance.

This is a strange job—people who aren't sick annoy you, and yet the really sick people are 'good jobs'. We are only happy when someone is suffering.

This feeling of only wanting 'good jobs' is one I keep wrestling with. It's not right to want people to suffer serious injury just so that I can have an 'interesting' day at work.

☕ HAPPINESS IS A WARM PIZZA

An excerpt from a conversation I just had with Control:

Control: 'Hello, EC50, we have a job for you'.

Me: 'Ah, you rotten buggers! I've just got myself a pizza'.

Control: 'Hold on a sec . . . OK, stand down (Other Callsign) is closer'.

Me: 'I love you like I have loved none other'.
Control: '. . . giggle, enjoy your pizza'.

Control can be nice sometimes . . . (*and if you want to do that again, I won't be complaining*).

☕ HOW TO BLOG AND NOT LOSE YOUR JOB

Listen to Uncle Reynolds as he sits you on his knee and explains these simple facts to stop you losing your job over blogging. These points relate mainly to work-blogs, but with a bit of thought will translate pretty well to anything that you write on the Internet. Most of this is just common-sense stuff, but there are people out there who falsely think that bloggers should be elevated over non-blogging employees.

Disclaimer—I am not an expert in employee law, I just have my opinions. Seek professional or union advice if you feel your job is under threat. At the end of the day, my company is trying to get fewer customers, not more. So my ideas may be a little screwed up. Don't come crying to me if you lose your job following my advice. Also don't come crying to me when I'm sitting on station trying to have a cup of tea.

How to blog, and not lose your job—version 1.0
You are not anonymous. In today's world of easy investigation (via the Internet of course) it is normally a matter of an hour's work to find out who a blogger is. It's really easy if the person who is doing the investigation works for the same company you do. Sure, you might use a pseudonym

and reduce your boss and fellow workers to nicknames, but it only takes one mention of some uncommon point to blow the whole thing open. For me, it was when I wrote about swallowing some HIV-positive blood; the news spread around 'in real life' and it didn't take a genius to work out who was writing my blog. In some places your company might be able to force your blog hosting company or ISP (Internet Service Provider) to reveal your details. *So write as if you are writing under your own name, or be honest and don't bother with a pseudonym.*

In a related note, you will probably be read by people who know you. It's probably inevitable, but folks who move in the same social circles as you will have similar interests. Your interest in blogging about your job in sheep shearing may well mean that when your colleague does a search for websites about sheep shearing for promotional interview reasons, your page may well turn up. If you are going to be publicising your blog, then there is a large chance that your target demographic will include some of your friends. Actually, if it doesn't then either your blog or your friendships are not very honest. *So blog as if everyone you know reads every word.*

You are not immune to the rule of law—really, you aren't. Blogging may be a great new thing, it may well have expanded quicker than any other medium in the history of humanity, but the laws of Libel, Slander and Defamation of Character (your country's laws may vary) still apply to you. Sure, the Internet fosters a sense of anonymity, and of free speech—but that only goes so far. A lot of bloggers who have been fired from their jobs have found out the hard way that you *can't* breach your company's rules/country's laws and expect the defence of 'But it was on the Internet' to hold much water. If I write something that defames someone, then they are fully within their rights to sue me, whether I'm published in a paper, a book or on the Internet. You have to follow civil and criminal laws online as well as offline. These will vary depending on where you live. For the Americans in the audience the whole 'Free Speech' bit in your constitution concerns your government making laws to curtail free speech, it says nothing about companies.

The truth will find you out—if you lie on your blog and there are any number of people reading then you will be found out. I'm not suggesting that there are a multitude of fact checkers out there, but it only needs one falsehood to completely blow any reputation you may have built up. If you lie about people then once again you are laying yourself open to a juicy bit of court action, which might bump up your pagehits, but not in a good way. If you aren't sure about a bit of information that you are writing about *mark such inconclusive evidence as being just that—inconclusive.*

If you think you will get in trouble with your blogging—ASK. I know that it may be easier to ask forgiveness than permission. But your company might be all out of forgiveness. If you think that your blogging might cause friction, or lead to you being disciplined, then ask your boss first. Go in prepared, with all the opinions and evidence that blogging is a good thing. Do a good enough job convincing them, and they might start paying you to blog. If they refuse flat out to let you blog, then consider whether this is a company you want to be working for, or if you want to blog strongly enough to risk losing your job. Do this, and don't be surprised when you get the sack.

Companies as well as people have secrets, and they will be mightily annoyed if those secrets are aired for everyone to look at. Companies have bigger secrets than individuals: they have to protect their profits, enjoy the support of their stockholders and maintain patent pending secrets. If you blab about 'Secret Project X', then the company will find some way to fire you. You might not think that revealing that chip X will be used in the new graphics card you are working on is proprietary information but it never hurts to check first. Just think before posting *'Who will this revealing secret hurt?'*: if you are not prepared to deal with the consequences, then don't post. Of course, if it is in the public interest to post about something, then you need to weigh up the possibility of being disciplined.

Companies, and people, have a reputation to protect: if you want to shout about how working in company X is like slavery (complete with whipping and a bread-and-water lunch programme), then that company might take a dislike to you doing so on the Internet. Actually, this is one of those things that is made worse because of the nature of the Internet. If you tell your wife that your job is awful, your company is unlikely to find out. Tell the same thing to a bunch of your friends down the pub and, if found out, the company may discipline you. Paint it in 6-foot high letters on the side of their building and you would expect to get the sack. Writing something on the Internet is much like painting it across the face of the moon. *If you are that unhappy, then find another job.* If you can't get another job, then at least be fairly subtle about your moaning. Your employers love you, and want what is best for you: if you are really that unhappy at work they will help you with some tough love by forcing you to choose other career options. You'll have to clear out your own desk though.

A lot of people won't like being written about—I mean, the Internet is full of freaks and weirdos right? Who'd want any details of their life on the 'inter-web super-info-highway' so just about anyone can read intimate details about them? If you are going to write about other people, then *anonymise them*. How you do this depends on the style of your blog; do you give them all nicknames, refer to them as initials or call them 'one of my workmates'? If you do give people nicknames, remember—they may well find out about it, and while calling your boss 'SmellyGit' may not be a sackable offence, it may well have a negative effect on your chances of a future promotion.

If work has a problem with your blog, find out exactly what the problem is, and work with them to correct it. Some workplaces won't let people blog at all, some have no policy for blogging, while others (perhaps most) have no idea what blogging is. Work with them to get a policy written, be

171

helpful, be cooperative and be evangelical. Telling your company that 'it isn't fair' when they ask you to stop your blog will work about as well as it did on your mother when you wanted to get that tattoo. Let them know how blogging 'humanises' the company, talk about how 'branding is a conversation'; let them know that you are performing 'grassroots, viral marketing'. If that doesn't work, let them know that people are going to start asking questions about why the blog has stopped, and that they will draw their own conclusions. This isn't a threat, but a reality. Get them to let you continue the blog but allow them to clear any information that you post about.

Can you blog on company time? Most companies have a policy about Internet usage. Your work might well have a policy that covers blogging without actually mentioning the word 'blog': probably something about using the Internet on company time. I suggest that if you are going to be posting during working hours you take a good long look at those policies. Remember, they are paying for you to work, not to write your diary (no matter how many people read it). Obviously, this doesn't apply to people whose job description is to blog. *If blogging is encroaching on your work or personal time in a negative way, then stop blogging—it's just not worth it.*

Sometimes blogging is just an excuse to get you fired. Sure, you might roll into work drunk, do very little work, backchat to your boss and fall asleep during the afternoon—but the reason they sacked you is because they found out you have a blog! I'm no expert on how easy it is to sack people, but I suspect that 'gross misconduct', 'failure to follow Internet policy', 'bringing the company into disrepute' and 'revealing company secrets' are fairly easy things to get past an industrial appeal board. I would imagine that some of the people who have been fired or disciplined have comforted themselves with the thought that 'it's because I have a blog, that's the only reason'. So be a good worker, then they won't be so quick to sack you.

Just because you blog, it doesn't make you special. Sure, you might have 10 000 page-hits a day, you are 'Slashdotted'. [Slashdotted (verb): to have your website linked to by the incredibly popular technology news website www.Slashdot.org.] This occasionally results in overwhelming levels of traffic, capable of knocking your website over on a regular basis, and you have Dave Weiner's [Don't ask!] home phone number—but that means nothing to your boss. Blogging doesn't bring with it a 'Get Out Of Jail Free' card, you have no 'Freedom of the Press', and just because thousands of people hang on your every word it doesn't mean that they will help you keep your job. Blogging grants you no immunity to normal disciplinary procedures. Sorry about that.

Does this emasculate your blog? Well, perhaps a little, but if you are posting inflammatory lies about people, revealing industrial secrets and whining about how much your job both 'sucks', and 'blows', then be fully prepared to be fired. If you are writing things that are really that negative, ask yourself if you are in the right job. Journalists working in countries under a dictator need to be careful about what they write—and while you might not get thrown in prison, or worse, just be aware that bad things happen to people who rock the boat. *It's not fair, but it's the way the world works.*

Finally, if you do lose your job, you have a whole audience of people finding out about it, any of which might help you get a job. I know at least two people (people I've met, not including people I've read about), who have gotten jobs based on their blogging. In most cases people are happier with their new jobs than their old, if only because their new company understands and supports their blogging.

FIT

Yesterday was busy, but busy in a good way in that most of the calls that I got actually warranted an ambulance. Actually, if I had been dropped on my head repeatedly as a child leading to me believing in the supernatural, I would have thought that there was something strange going on. The majority of my jobs, and a lot of the jobs that I heard being given out over the radio, were for people having seizures.

The first call of the day was to a known epileptic who had been fitting while in the bath. Luckily, his father heard him thrashing against the side of the bath and pulled him out before he could drown. He was still quite drowsy, confused and a bit 'punchy'—normal for people who have just finished having a fit. The ambulance crew got there

174

and as the patient was a known epileptic, and was feeling better, he was left at home with the instruction that should he have another fit, then he should go to hospital.

I then bounced from that job to another young male who was having recurrent epileptic fits: in over an hour he hadn't managed to recover from a fit. He had three fits and was still extremely 'floppy'. The crew asked for my help in controlling him in the back of the ambulance, so I left the car and helped keep his airway clear while we 'blued' him into the local hospital. He had one more fit in the back of the ambulance, which I never like dealing with, as there are a few too many hard surfaces in the back of an ambulance that you can injure yourself on.

The ambulance crew then returned me to my car, and I was pleasantly surprised to discover that it was still there, and that the wheels were still attached.

I then ended up going back to my first epileptic, as he had suffered another seizure. This time the ambulance crew took him to hospital for a check-up. There are a couple of things that can reduce the effectiveness of antiepileptic medication, and while the patient's family believed that he had been drinking recently, it is always a good idea to rule out the other causes for an increase in seizure frequency.

Then there was a hoax call for a 'pedestrian versus car', which had me, the HEMS doctors, an ambulance and the police trying in vain to find a victim. Great . . .

Next was a middle-aged man, who was having his first heart attack. The call was given as a chest pain.

When I walked in the room and saw how ashen he was, I immediately broke out the oxygen and medication. He gave a classic history and description of a heart attack; luckily, the ambulance was quick in turning up and the job went like clockwork, with the patient getting transported to hospital very quickly.

Then I went to a patient with cancer of the bowel who had abdominal pain; an easy job in one way, but rather shocking in another because the patient was the same age as me . . .

My final (late) job was to a 1-year-old child who had been . . . wait for it . . . fitting—the very common febrile fit (when a child has a temperature that rises quickly they can often have a seizure). While it is a medical emergency, it's something that because we deal with them a lot we find an 'easy job'. Essentially, you cool the child down, and give them oxygen.

In more general news, the sat-nav screen on one of our ambulances was stolen the other night. Someone broke into the ambulance to steal a bit of equipment that helps the community. It says it all for some of the people in this area really . . .

🚑 45+

Yesterday was fairly busy, but the two remarkable jobs of the day were caused by what we in the trade call 'Tricky extrication'.

The first job was to a young male collapsed in a bookmaker's toilet. I've been to a couple of these, and for some reason bookmakers' toilets are favoured places for junkies to 'shoot up' in. I've

176

been to more junkies in bookmakers' than I have drunks in pub toilets. Do not ask me why.

The toilet itself was 3 feet by 5 feet, and in it was a heavily drunken Lithuanian, covered in vomit, urine and the drink of champions—'White Lightning', about 3 litres' worth. He was, to all intents, unconscious—unable to talk, stand, walk or do anything except drool . . . and he drooled a lot.

Because of the size of the toilet (barely enough room for one person, let alone me as well), the slippery floor (vomit, urine and cheap, nasty cider) and the state of the patient (big, thickset, heavy and completely unable to help) I had to grab him by his belt buckles, and with the aid of the crew manhandle him out to the ambulance.

I followed the crew to the hospital, so that I could wash some of the 'stuff' I had all over my arms—the hospital knew the patient, because he had been there yesterday, for exactly the same thing . . .

The last job of the day was to a 45-stone male (285 kg for the metrically minded) with difficulty in breathing. He was up one flight of stairs, found it very difficult to walk, and was in a flat full of cardboard boxes. It took us an hour to get him out of the house, down the stairs and into the ambulance and at the hospital it took another half an hour to get him inside. Our trolley-bed (and these are the new trolley-beds—fairly strong things) was buckling under his weight, and there was a moment or two when I thought it would collapse under the weight.

It took so long to get him out of the house that I got an hour's worth of overtime—which, for my mercenary nature, was rather nice.

RETURN JOB

I could hardly believe it, the first job of my shift was to the 45+ stone patient who was my last job on my last shift.

It only took 45 minutes to get him out of his flat this time, which just goes to prove that practice does indeed make perfect.

I've been back to him twice more. He's a nice enough person, but I still dread the call to his flat.

HOAXES

One of my regular readers is someone from an Ambulance Control: they left the following in my comments section about why we on the road tend not to see too many hoax calls.

We do get a fair number of hoax calls in Control. Most of them can be spotted a mile off, however, and consist of someone under the age of 16 requesting police, fire and ambulance for some unfeasible event. They usually hang up when you read them back the address they are calling from or, if they are in a call box (which they usually are), tell them to 'look up at the security camera in the box so I can see your face' or 'the doors of the phone box will now lock automatically—the police are on their way to catch you for making NAUGHTY HOAX CALLS'. Obviously, you have to be 100% sure that it is a hoax before you do this, otherwise someone will die and then you will get the sack.

I also spend a fair deal of time when working on the dispatch desks calling back suspected hoaxes from call boxes until a member of the public answers and confirms there are no dying individuals lying around that we ought to be attending to.

One or two do slip through the net, though. There was an almighty ruckus when some really 'funny' people decided to tell us that someone had fallen down the stairs and then given birth to her sixth baby on the spot. A whole fleet of ambulances and midwives turned up to find a bunch of sniggering teenagers on the doorstep and no sign of any woman or baby. They didn't even have the sense to give a false address. One of the midwives rang up and shouted at me for half an hour.

So, thanks to the folks up in Control around the country for dealing with the obvious hoax calls.

MASKING HISTORIES

Sometimes patients can be awkward buggers: all their signs and symptoms point to one illness, and it is only a bit later, with a bit more investigation, that you find out what is actually wrong with them.

Today was a case in point: I got called to a 42-year-old male who had been suffering from chest pain for the past 2 hours. I turned up and started my examination of him. He had fallen down the stairs the day before, his chest was painful when I pushed on it and he had no symptoms leading me to believe that the problem was anything to do with his heart. I immediately thought that the pain was muscular in nature, rather than a more serious cardiac problem.

The only thing was that his pulse felt 'funny', a strange little 'thrumming' sensation that was a little like a double heartbeat. I thought that if I hooked

179

him up to my cardiac monitor I'd have a better idea what was going on. However, the leads on the monitor weren't working so I would have to wait until the ambulance turned up.

It was a little embarrassing because the patient and his wife were both doctors (probably working in research). Both were happy with their treatment and the ambulance soon turned up. The patient was connected to their monitor and we found out that he was in SVT (supraventricular tachycardia) which is a rhythm problem with the heart, causing it to beat too quickly.

The actual 'chest pain' was probably related to the fall, being either a bruise or a muscle strain, while the patient's real problem was hidden from a cursory examination. It is only because we have the capability to electrically examine the heart that the patient was sped into hospital rather than taken in normally.

I'm wondering if the fall somehow caused the arrhythmia, it's probably not outside the realms of possibility.

Knowing what the patient's problem was also meant that the ambulance crew didn't look embarrassed after handing the patient over to the nurses at the hospital.

Tomorrow I have a special learning day—learning how to 'maintain personal safety', how to defuse aggressive situations and how to escape from grapples and the like . . .

I went to this patient about 9 months later. He'd had a sudden cardiac arrest and, despite our best efforts, he died.

🚑 CARROTS

As promised, the quality of this blog is about to nosedive, as I discuss some of the things I have personally witnessed up a patient's rectum.

I've not seen a FBUA (foreign body up arse) while in the ambulance service—I think most people are so embarrassed that they tend to make their own way to hospital rather than risk being laughed at by two hairyarmed ambulance people.

The one that sticks most in my mind was the first one I ever came across. I was working in A&E at the time, and I think I'd only been there a year or so, when I saw a load of doctors crouched around an abdominal X-ray.

'You can see it there', said one.

'Don't be daft, but you *can* see the bowel being pushed out of shape', another said dismissively.

'Of course you can't see it', said another, 'It's organic . . .'

Being a nosey nurse I asked what they were looking at, and was told that the patient had a carrot up their rectum. Looking closely at the X-ray I could see where the lower part of the bowel was *stretched* upward by a large amount. There was no sign of the alleged carrot, but then it wouldn't show up in a normal X-ray film anyway, it being as organic as the flesh that X-rays go through unimpeded.

The story I was told was that the patient was a 72-year-old male who had gotten his groceries and was taking a short-cut across the local park when he was 'caught short'. Desperate to open his bowels, he had dropped his trousers and crouched behind a tree to—cough—'have a poo'. However,

181

two 15-year-old boys ran up behind him, grabbed a carrot from the bag and inserted it rectally.

The patient didn't want the police involved because he 'didn't want to be any trouble'.

Us professionally trained staff were of course sympathetic to his plight, and obviously believed every word of his tale.

Who am I kidding . . . we didn't believe a word of it. The patient went to have the carrot surgically removed and all was well in the world.

Carrots are a popular thing for FBUA—it was a year or two later, when I had become much more cynical, that I came across another 'carrot insertion incident'. The patient was a young male who fully admitted having taken some 'Ecstasy', and had been fooling around with a carrot when it had become stuck.

The patient himself wasn't too bothered because, ever mindful of disease, he had put a condom on the carrot.

So, I think the government is giving our youths the wrong message when it tries to dissuade drug use. Instead of the dangers of overdose, heart attacks and reduced sexual function, they should just show a picture of someone putting a condom-wrapped carrot up their arse while thinking it's a good idea.

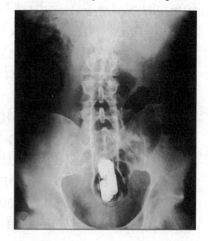

It's not all carrots, as some people have already mentioned in the comments section, sometimes it can be things that are 'supposed' (sort of) to be used in such ways.

I was working in triage in A&E at the time, where my role was to do the initial patient assessment to see how urgently they needed to be seen. A young man and his girlfriend walked in, the male was in obvious distress and I soon found out why.

The pair had been indulging in 'sex games' and they had been using a vibrator. Unfortunately for the male, his girlfriend had gotten a bit vigorous in inserting it into her boyfriend's rectum, and it had been sucked into his body.

What people need to realise is that there can often be a 'suction effect', which means that things will just shoot up there and refuse to come out.

Well, being the kind of nurse I once was—I had to have a listen. So the stethoscope came out, and after being gently applied to his abdomen I could hear a loud buzzing noise. I wondered how long the batteries would last.

The patient, while worried about his health, was more concerned that his mum would find out that he was at the hospital, and would turn up demanding to know what had happened to her son. Not wanting to be the nurse who had to explain to an irate mother that her son had a vibrator stuck up his arse, I got him seen as quickly as possible.

We got an X-ray taken—you could see the circuitry really well, but the 'body' of the vibrator was a lot harder to see.

He was booked for surgery, and just before he was about to go the theatres his mum turned up.

He started off by trying to tell her that he had a generic abdominal pain, but she questioned why he needed to go to surgery for a belly-ache. So he sat her down in a private room (provided by me, I may

183

be cruel, but I'm not *that* cruel) and explained exactly what happened.

To be fair, his mum took it quite well, there was no shouting, ranting, arguing or even sniggering. Instead she was supportive, if a little bemused.

If it was me I think my mum would disown me . . .

The vibrator was removed under anaesthetic, and the patient made a full recovery.

I don't know what happened to the vibrator though . . .

I posted a couple other stories about FBUA. It was all I wrote about for a week. Lots of people liked the stories. As I have mentioned earlier these are the sorts of stories you tell down the pub and people will end up buying you drinks.

DOORKNOB

For the final post about FBUA (for I am on night-shifts from tonight), I'd like to relate the tale of the doorknob.

A 45-year-old male came into A&E with a doorknob inserted where the sun doesn't shine.

His story was less than original. Apparently he enjoyed vacuuming his house while naked. While doing this he had backed up against his living room door, only to have the doorknob disappear up his rectum. Unfortunately, the doorknob was loose, and when he tried to remove himself, the doorknob gave way and thus became trapped up his bum. Thankfully, he got dressed *before* making his way to hospital.

Cue surgery, and removal of said object, when asked if it caused much damage, the surgeon replied '*It rect'um*'.

. . . Bad joke, I know, but that's surgeons for you—she probably spent the entire surgery thinking that one up.

I vaguely remember two other stories: one of a woman who came to our hospital with a bed-knob inserted anally. The other is of a person who shaves doll heads, swallows them and then gains sexual gratification from passing them in his stool. This may not be true (I read it on the Internet), but it wouldn't surprise me if it were.

SHORT-TERM MEMORY LOSS

I've just come back from a 'Matern-a-taxi', and it always amuses me when I turn up *5 minutes* after they have called for an ambulance. Then, when I knock on the door, they look out the window, take in the uniform, the ambulance parked outside, and the big bag of medical equipment and ask . . .

'Who is it?'

LIARS

I'm kind of prosaic about our regular callers, they have chronic conditions (normally brought on by drinking), but they are normally easy to deal with and, if you keep friendly with them, they are seldom trouble.

. . . Until they start being incontinent on the back of your ambulance. But that is a subject for another day.

What I do dislike are the regulars who feel the

185

need to lie to our call-takers.

Take regular patient number one: she calls for an ambulance, claiming that she has had a fit. When I turn up (I get mobilised for patients having fits a lot), she tells us that she hasn't had a fit, but her legs hurt, so can we take her to the hospital. Repeat this once or twice a day and you wonder why some of us won't be too upset when we eventually find her dead in the gutter.

Tonight I went to regular patient number two: he is an alcoholic, who tonight told our Control that he had been assaulted 20 minutes earlier and had had a seizure as a result of this assault. I get sent the job, and speed 3 miles to get to the patient, only to find him drunk; he hadn't been assaulted and there was no evidence that he had been fitting.

It isn't the actual going to the patient that bothers me, as I mentioned earlier, it's an easy job. What does annoy me is that I rush to these calls, putting myself and other road users at risk, only to find the patient not undergoing a life-threatening event. I get very cynical about these jobs.

I've tried telling them that if they call for an ambulance and say they have a painful leg, then they will still get an ambulance, but that they won't be putting other peoples lives at risk by having me drive on blue lights and sirens (at risk of hitting a pedestrian), or by taking an ambulance away from someone who urgently needs an ambulance at that time.

But still they insist on calling for an ambulance with phantom illnesses.

The woman that I mention as regular caller number one, has been found a place to live in a nunnery. We haven't heard from her since.

🚐 *CAN'T* TOUCH HER

My shift ends at 6:30 in the morning, so I was very happy to be left alone from 11 p.m.

Except that at *6:20* I get a job (I ask them if they are joking—they aren't). The job is a chest pain on a bus, in a bus garage.

It is also so far out my normal area that I have to study the map for some time before I can work out how to get there.

I turn up to find out that the 'patient' is an alcoholic who is asleep in one of the buses. She denies any chest pain, injury or illness and after some persuasion she leaves the bus under her own power and leaves the scene.

If I were being cynical, I would be thinking that the bus company, unable to actually touch her for fear of assault, has called for an ambulance purely so that someone else is responsible for getting her off the bus.

Previous experience would suggest that this is indeed the case.

Why would they say she had chest pain—perhaps they know that this gets the quickest response from us . . .

Oh well . . . it's all overtime.

🚐 HAI

One of the bugbears that each political party is addressing for the upcoming election is the concept of HAIs (hospital-acquired infections). So far, the politicians have been mainly concentrating on MRSA (methicillinresistant *Staphylococcus aureus*), but this is not the only thing that you can catch in hospital.

I've just come from a job where a 95-year-old female, who had spent a week in hospital for a blood clot on the leg, was suffering from some difficulty in breathing.

The patient had been discharged from the local hospital yesterday, and during the night had developed laboured breathing, a cough and a feeling of tightness in the chest.

Upon examination it seemed that the pain was not related to any cardiac cause. The tightness was worse when she breathed in, she had a slight temperature and, coupled with the cough and no history of heart problems, it seemed like a simple chest infection.

The patient and her daughter were happy with this provisional diagnosis, but were glad that she would be going to hospital for some more tests.

. . . But then the daughter asked me where her mother could have caught her chest infection . . . and I really didn't want to say 'from the hospital'.

I imagine that the ward from which the patient had been discharged had one or more people with a chest infection. Having worked in a hospital I know that a lot of patients, and their visitors, don't cover their mouths when they cough, and it seems completely reasonable that this is where the patient caught this infection.

It is probably unrelated to nurse or doctor hygiene (as these sorts of infection are often airborne) but instead caused by something as simple as someone not covering their mouth when coughing. It might not have been another patient— hospital wards see a lot of visitors, including small children who are constantly exposed to, and incubating, infections.

It seems to me that a lot of hospital infections could be cut if patient visitors didn't treat the ward like some form of hotel, tracking their infections in and out of the community, and generally acting as if the rules of hygiene don't apply to them. I'm a big fan of restricted visiting for the majority of cases—and is there really any reason for children to be dragged around a hospital at all hours of the day?

It used to drive me barmy when I was running a ward.

However, medical staff do indeed need to improve their hand washing.

🚑 FLAT

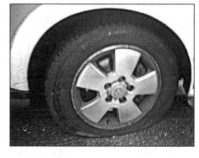

So there I was, pulling up to a job (male fitting in street), the ambulance was already there (having been dispatched from the same station as me, only 2 minutes earlier).

Then I heard a loud bang, and thought the bottom had dropped off the car—the crew on scene and the police who were there all looked in my direction.

My front tyre had burst as I had ridden up the kerb a little too forcefully.

There I was, stuck by the side of the road waiting for the tyre fitter to come and change my tyre. I may well have a spare tyre in the back of the car, but if I fit it, and it later falls off, then I'm to blame.

I returned to station to find a new wallpaper on the station computer . . .

'Brand new tyre required for Vauxhall Astra FRU, All enquiries to J2 station c/o Tom Reynolds'.

I love my workmates . . .

DENTIST

I often moan about GPs that leave their patients who are seriously ill alone in their waiting rooms, or outside in the street having a cigarette. But until today I'd never been to a dentist (which might explain the state of my teeth—*ho-ho*).

The patient was a 42-year-old female who was 'shaking' on the dentist's chair. I arrived and the patient was still in the chair, and was being given oxygen and reassurance by the dentist.

The patient had a long history of these episodes, and the dentist gave me a complete handover, including the social history of the patient, and while I was assessing the patient was still spending time reassuring her. The patient was not suffering from anything serious, but she agreed to go to the hospital for a quick check-up.

I must admit I was really impressed by this dentist for actually caring for their patient. It is only as I sit writing this that I realise that I'm impressed at a health-care professional that is *actually doing their job.*

Isn't that sad . . .

🚑 RADIATING PAIN

Sometimes you are really glad the patient isn't facing you.

I went to an elderly male with 'chest pain'; the ambulance crew turned up at pretty much the same time, so I found myself standing behind the patient as they got a history from him.

'Where is the pain?', the ambulance attendant asked.

'Here', he replied pointing to the top of his chest.

'What does the pain feel like?'

'Kind of a burning pain'.

'Does the pain go anywhere else?'

'Well, it didn't go with me to my friends house . . .'

. . . Cue me trying (thankfully successfully) to stop from laughing out loud. Instead, I managed to restrain myself to just some silent sniggering.

For those that aren't aware, chest pain which is related to the heart often radiates to the jaw or arm.

Bless him, I love this job.

I've just spoken to the crew, and the pain was related to his heart.

🚑 VALUES

I was called to a 39-year-old male, possibly dead. As I entered the house I saw his relatives crying, and sitting on a kitchen chair was my patient. He looked dead and wasn't breathing.

I felt for a pulse, didn't feel one, so I hooked up the heart monitor and there was no electrical activity at all.

I turned around to his relatives and told them that there was nothing that I could do for him, and that an ambulance crew would turn up shortly to help them out.

It took 10 minutes for the crew to turn up, and I didn't recognise them at all—they must have come from outside our area.

Suddenly, one of the crew said they had felt a pulse!

The patient was also breathing. Oxygen was given and he was rushed out to the ambulance. All that was running through my head was how I had 'starved' him of oxygen, and how much trouble I was going to be in.

One of the crew told me to fake my paperwork, and say that I'd given the patient oxygen. But I knew I was going to get into trouble.

I felt sick for the patient, and sick for myself. This is the sort of mistake that can cost you your job . . .

. . . Then the postman rang my doorbell, and I woke up from the nightmare I was having.

It's funny how this job can play on your mind—the things that I've seen and dealt with on this job and as an A&E nurse. Yet, it seems that the fear of making a mistake with a patient is still the thing that scares me most.

I've dealt with murders, mutilations and miscarriages. I've seen death in the faces of 3-month-old children, 14-year-old girls and 22-year-old men. I've dealt with limbs hanging off, distraught relatives and people vomiting blood until they die.

But the only thing that haunts my dreams is the

fear of doing something wrong.

Shouldn't the patient have more of a place in my mind?

🚑 ROUGH

Today is one of those days where I really need to be careful, otherwise the disjunction between what the public expects of us and what we actually do will get me in trouble.

At the moment my body is feeling ready to give up, a troublesome changeover from night to day work doesn't help; neither does the sore throat or the feeling that my soul is still on holiday in Seattle and waiting for a flight back to my body in London.

This means that the chances of me having a 'sense of humour' failure are greater than normal.

I noticed it yesterday with my last job—I was called to a '60-year-old male, collapsed in park'. Now there are of course many reasons why someone collapses in the park, and while I keep an open mind the chances are very high that it is alcohol related.

So I got there, and there was a concerned member of the public fussing over a drunk alcoholic. All power to him, he had spotted someone in distress and was trying to help out as best he could, and I'd much rather have people like that compared with the calls we get of 'Man lying in street, poss. dead. Caller cannot stay on scene', which *always* seems to be a drunk.

The care I gave was the same as the care I would normally give, but I wasn't as 'warm' as I normally am. I was polite, but there was something deep down in me that really couldn't be bothered with dealing with yet another alcoholic.

The ambulance turned up about a minute later, and took care of the patient—but I was aware that the bystander was probably not happy with my apparent lack of empathy.

This is that disjunction that I mentioned: the public expects us to be constantly caring people, dealing with what they see as a serious emergency, while to us it is a regular alcoholic, with very little newly wrong with them. While we often hide our apathy behind our professionalism, it can sometimes slip.

It's that sort of job that will earn you a complaint from someone for being 'not caring enough'.

The fact that I feel rough (through no fault of my own) might just mean that the mask of caring might slip—and while I have no problem with people who are actually ill, if I get the usual rubbish, I'll have to be very, very careful.

I never did get a complaint about this job and it shouldn't surprise people that us ambulance staff are human too, and that we have our 'off' days as well.

WHETHER THE WEATHER

One of my commenters asked if it was true that the full moon affected people so much that the local hospital had to hire extra night staff every month. There have been scientific studies to disprove this, and I have never worked in a hospital that hired extra staff on the basis of the phases of the moon.

But it did get me thinking about the effects that the weather has upon people, because in my experience this *does* have an appreciable effect.

When I was teaching children, we would dread days when it was windy, because we knew that the children would be more active and more prone to be disobedient. Another of my commenters said exactly the same thing, so I know it wasn't a local phenomenon.

It works for adults too. I'm much busier on windy days, and while this is just my impression, I always seem to think that there are also many more assaults.

If the weather is grey and overcast, we tend to go to more old folk who are sitting indoors, or more commonly, falling over indoors. Sometimes you get the impression that they just want someone to talk to—or to not be alone. There also seem to be more suicide attempts as well, and it is fairly well known that suicide rates go up in springtime. So, on those rainy spring days you end up seeing a lot of paracetamol overdoses.

Spring and autumn rains (and in England, summer rains) bring with them car-versus-car collisions, as an infrequent rain lifts off the layer of rubber and pollution left on the road by passing cars and the roads become a skid pan. Fallen leaves on the road don't help, and neither do the effects of the rapidly changing hours of daylight on a driver's body clock.

Ice on the streets means that we will be going to plenty of 'Nan Down!' calls—little old ladies falling over. When working in the hospitals I remember one icy day where I personally dealt with **23** elderly people with broken wrists caused by falling on the ice.

When the weather is sunny there can also be

chaos on the streets—this Sunday had really nice, sunny weather, the kind of weather you only seem to remember from your childhood. East London has a lot of narrow residential streets, with cars parked nose to tail on both sides of the road. If these streets are 'quiet' then children tend to forget that cars do occasionally travel down them (thankfully not often at any speed).

So, this Sunday there were more than the usual number of children being hit by cars, I went to one where a 6-year-old had run out between two parked cars and been struck. He had a minor head wound, and complained of neck pain, so I put a hard collar on him and when the ambulance crew turned up we did a full restraint. He was an excellent patient—normally I can't stand kids, but he was exceptionally brave, and when I explained about the collar, he was happy to have it on because he had seen them in use on the television.

There was also a (well behaved) crowd of about 30 people standing around, and when the police turned up they got the people out the way by saying 'I know it's a cliché but, please move along there is nothing to see . . .'

It's a good job I don't get performance anxiety.

The hot weather also brings out the people who start drinking at lunchtime and continue throughout the day; tie this in with a lot of sporting fixtures and we find ourselves going to a lot of fights in a lot of pubs.

A strange thing happened tonight.

For the first time ever, I was 'recognised'.

The job itself was simple enough, genuine illness that had become worse. I walked into the house had a quick assessment of the situation, and then said my usual bit which goes something like . . .

'OK, I'm the fast car, so I turn up to make sure everyone is still breathing. There will be an ambulance along in a bit to actually take you to hospital'.

I *wasn't* expecting one of the relatives to then say.

'You also blog about it as well—I recognise your face'.

Sudden panic, followed by an admission that I was indeed that particular ambulance person.

It's strange, I suppose I've always thought that this might happen one day, although given the amount of alcoholics I see, and the way that they don't tend to read blogs, I thought that it might take longer than it has.

It's not as if I altered my treatment in any way, and if anything it made the treatment easier, as he knew that I wasn't some fly-by-night cowboy.

I hope . . .

The person who recognised me left a comment on the blog saying that they were happy with the treatment they received. Apparently I have been recognised at least once more, but that the person involved didn't want to admit it to me. Apart from these two times I remain blissfully anonymous.

🚐 DECOMP

For the first time in ages I got sent to a decomposing body. The social housing people had been around the elderly gentleman's flat a week earlier, noticed a bit of a smell, but ignored it. When they came back a week later and the smell was still there they decided to talk to the caretakers. The caretakers beat down the door—looked at what was in the bedroom and called the police.

The police then passed the job on to us, so that we could confirm death.

The first thing that you notice when dealing with a 'decomp' is the smell, it's quite unlike anything else—it settles in the back of the throat and stays there for some time. I was sucking mints and drinking tea for some time after leaving the flat to try and get the *taste* out of my mouth.

The other thing is the flies. You find yourself in a room with flies that have grown and fed on the tissues of a dead person. Sometimes they land on you. For hours afterwards you can feel them crawling on your skin (I can still feel them now, about 8 hours later). It doesn't make me feel dirty, but it does make me scratch.

The sight of the corpse isn't too bad after all that. The eyes are gone, and the skin is either dark brown or black. The thing that makes you realise that the thing in front of you was once alive is the hair. The hair is the same as when the person died, in this case it was white, clean and neatly brushed. The entry points to the body (the eyes, the nose and mouth) are crawling with flies and maggots, and this is the only movement you'll see.

198

The patient looked to have died in his sleep. He was lying in his bed and it looked as if he had simply passed away without waking. Not a bad way to go.

I can see this being my end, as I plan to outlive all my relatives, I don't talk to my neighbours at the moment (because, in part, they don't speak English) and at the rate I'm going I doubt I'll be married.

I hope I make a *really* stinky corpse. Perhaps making a young trainee EMT vomit in disgust, so that everyone at their station can have a good laugh at their expense.

Yes, since you ask, us ambulance people tend to have a strange sense of humour.

🚑 MATERN-A-WATER-TAXIS

The other interesting job yesterday (for, with one exception, today was a day full of maternities and elderly chest pains) was a maternity with a difference. The patient was supposed to have a home delivery, but the delivery was taking too long, the mother was getting tired and the baby had meconium-stained amniotic fluid. Meconium is babies' first poo. It's a sign of a baby being in some distress.

The midwives decided that it would be better if the baby was delivered in hospital, so called for an ambulance to transport the mother.

What was different was that the patient lived on a houseboat.

. . . Cue myself, carrying a load of heavy, expensive equipment down narrow docks,

199

narrower walkways and unbelievably narrow boat walkway, then out again carrying even more of the midwife's equipment.

🚑 LITTLE THINGS

First off, there is an emergency GP doing the rounds who seems to have some strange ideas. Examples of his work are the elderly woman who is dizzy and has jaundice, a man with all-over muscle pain for 2 weeks and an elderly man with 'fluid on the lungs'. All these were prescribed antibiotics and were told, 'It's probably an infection, but I don't know where'. I'm not sure if its the same GP, but if it is, then they really are clueless.

This is probably why the Primary Care Trusts like the ambulance service—because we don't faff around, but take everyone who is ill to hospital, and leave the well ones at home.

I went to a little old lady who had fainted. Absolute darling (if only because she laughed at my 'you should take more water with your gin if it makes you dizzy' joke), but who didn't want to go to hospital because she cares for her disabled husband. They lived in a warden-controlled flat, but the wardens in those places are not supposed to do any 'caring' work. Our patient wouldn't go to hospital and leave her husband, so, falling back on my nursing experience, I got Control to call the social services that look after that family. After promising that everything would be fine, she agreed to go to hospital.

Why did I go through Control to contact the social workers, rather than phone them myself?

Well . . . (*as mentioned previously*) Control record all the phone calls they make, so if someone promises to do something, then we have the proof . . .

. . . *Not that I have a lot of experience dealing with social workers at all* . . .

I got a job as a '15-year-old Suspended at school' (suspended is a polite way of saying 'dead'), I don't think my foot lifted off the accelerator pedal at all to the school, and I suspect that a lot of rubber was left on the pavement as I power-slid around the corners (who says computer racing games are no use?). I hit the school at about the same time as the ambulance crew (who had also driven like maniacs), and we ran up three flights of stairs, across the school, and down three flights of stairs. I saw the girl lying on her side, rolled her over, and had a huge sigh of relief as she recoiled in horror from my ugly face staring down at her.

The patient had very little wrong with her, much to our relief.

We were all understandably happy, but then the adrenaline crash hit us pretty hard, and coupled with the physical exertion of running, I felt like crap for half an hour, until a nice cup of tea worked its magic.

However . . .

Tomorrow, I shall be on the hunt: I shall be hunting for a specific lollipop man (or whatever they are called these days). When I find him, I shall be shoving his stick where the sun doesn't shine.

The reason?

Picture the scene—I'm racing down the road on lights and sirens, and since I think that I'm going to a dead 15-year-old, I'm driving, as previously mentioned, at a stupidly fast speed.

. . . So what does this bloody idiot do to a kid waiting on the other side of the road? He tries to get the kid to run across the road before I get there!

This sort of thing makes me want to go stabby . . .

Lots of things make me want to go stabby, but this guy took the prize for sheer stupidity. Despite looking for him for the rest of the week I never did find him.

🚐 A HAPPY JOB (FOR A CHANGE)

Barely 2 days since moaning about Matern-a-taxis, than I get sent to another one.

'We have a job for you', said Control.

'Of course you do, I was just about to have a cup of tea', I replied, 'so . . . what is it'.

I looked at the display terminal in the car.

'It's a bloody maternity', I was outraged, 'One-minute contractions—I bet they'll be 10 minutes apart when I get there'.

'I reckon they will as well', replied Control.

So I dutifully shot down there, to a place fairly well known to me—it's a large housing unit for teenagers; they all have social workers and are looked after pretty well. To be honest I think it's a pretty good place, I've never had any trouble there and the residents get a fair bit of support.

I entered the accommodation, to find a young woman having a contraction while standing in a puddle of fluid.

No problem, I thought, the waters have just broken.

'I really want to go a poo', she said.

'Oh bugger', thought me.

202

It's one of the guides as to how close you are to delivering the baby—if you want to go poo, then birth probably isn't too far away.

Then she had another strong contraction, then another—they were 1 minute apart . . .

So I turned on my breezy, 'relax, everything is fine, nothing to worry about' personality and quickly phoned Control to see where the ambulance was. I was told it was on its way and they turned up pretty quickly, but by then birth was too close, so we decided to 'stay and play'.

A midwife was called for, and she told Control she would make her way there in her own car. I do have a slight problem with this. If an ambulance crew needs a midwife, it's generally as an emergency, otherwise we transport the patient to hospital. If it's an emergency then shouldn't we pick up the midwife and get her to the job on blue lights and sirens?

The ambulance paramedic and I let the ambulance EMT do most of the mucky work. Not because we are (particularly) cruel, but because it was his first ambulance delivery . . . and it's a good experience.

A lovely baby girl was born at 10:29, and we let the father cut the umbilical cord.

Then, after all the screaming, poo, blood, fluid and pain, the midwife turned up.

Luckily for us the birth was uncomplicated. It took maybe a shade longer than I like, and apparently the birth fluid was stained green (to my eyes it looked normal, but then I do have strong prescription glasses). The fluid being green means that the baby may have pooed while being born, and that could be a sign of distress.

I also managed to use all my bad jokes during the delivery, which is a sign of how long the delivery took, because I have a lot of bad jokes.

It's always good to be involved in the birth of a baby: everyone is happy, you hopefully end up with a pretty little baby, and dad normally bounds around taking photos of everything. It always feels like a 'job well done'.

We don't get much training with birthing, and when we do deliver it's normally in an awkward place, with poor lighting and loads of people panicking. It would be nice if our training encompassed a little time in a maternity unit, rather than sitting in a classroom for a morning.

However, in an uncomplicated birth, it really is a case of just catching them as they pop out.

Anyway, it gave me a big grin on my face for the next few hours.

🚑 PHYSICIAN RESPONSE UNIT

The PRU is a doctor and paramedic team who run from the Royal London hospital. Their role is to see patients who might not need a trip to hospital, and to treat them at home—thus saving the patient having to wait around in A&E for a couple of hours, and freeing up emergency services for more serious cases. They also provide support for more serious incidents where a doctor on scene is a really good idea.

I've had a couple of jobs with them; normally it's something simple like a patient with a chest infection or other minor illness. A lot of patients in our area don't have a GP to see them, and so A&E

and the ambulance service is their first, and only, port of call.

The PRU is manned by a doctor and a paramedic; they drive around in a blue Subaru that was donated by a firm of solicitors.

The last time I saw their statistics, they managed to treat a patient at home without needing an ambulance, or a hospital visit, 30–40% of the time.

(They also wear the orange HEMS jumpsuits for some strange reason . . .)

I mention them because I had a job with them the other day. I was called to a little old lady who had collapsed in the street. I got there first, and started my assessment—she was frail-looking, but fully aware of what was happening to her. Her pulse was on the low side of normal, and her blood pressure felt a little low (just off the pulse), then, just as I'm about to check her blood pressure using our normal tools, the PRU rolled up behind me and three orange-clad people jumped out.

I gave a quick handover to the doctor, and he continued assessing the patient while I measured her blood sugar. Her blood sugar was normal, but her blood pressure was pretty low; a quick look at her heart rhythm didn't show anything unusual, and neither did a further physical examination.

Meanwhile we were waiting for an ambulance.

I was asked if I wanted to cannulate the patient (put a needle in a vein so that drugs or fluids could be given), but as it's been 3 years since I last cannulated someone, and she was a nice little old lady (instead of some stinky obnoxious drunk) I declined—I'm not *that* cruel to inflict my rusty skills on someone who is actually nice for a change . . .

There was still no ambulance to send, so it was decided to take the patient to the hospital in the back of the Subaru as the patient wasn't getting the investigations she needed lying around the local market. All I can say, is that she looked a lot healthier sitting in the back of the car, than lying on a market bench.

The PRU (when it is running, manning the vehicle is apparently a bit of a nightmare) is a quality addition to the local NHS, and someone has definitely taught the doctors how to be nice to ambulance crews. It's just a shame that the Royal London doesn't get any extra money to run this service, which covers the gaps in local GP provisioning.

Just one more bit of the NHS being run on goodwill and charity . . .

☕ NOWT

No jobs yet. I have a suspicion that although I have told Control that I am working, they may have forgotten to put me on the main computer.

So my options are as follows . . ..

(1) Sit on station, have something to eat, have a sleep and if they continue to ignore me, have a restful night.

(2) Let guilt get the better of me, give Control a ring and then spend the rest of my night actually working . . .

Guess I'm going to be phoning Control then . . .

This happened a couple of times, and each time I reminded them that I was working. It only took 4 months for them to start remembering me.

206

🚐 TESCO

I've just gotten some milk for the station, and chocolate (and some other, healthier foodstuffs) to see me through the night.

I've got to say, I love the way people doing their shopping stare as I walk past them in my uniform, clutching a shopping basket.

Not that I enjoy being the centre of attention, but the looks I get make me think that people are *disappointed* that us medical emergency types actually eat.

Try working a 12-hour shift without eating and I think you'd find yourself a bit less able to deal with the stresses of the job.

A happy belly equals a happy EMT.

Seriously. Keep us fed and watered and we'll be quite happy to tackle anything you can throw at us. Starving ambulance crews get a bit . . . 'testy'.

🚐 SCUM

So a crew (not me, I'm relaxing on station) get called to a woman who is 38 weeks pregnant and has been mugged.

Her mobile phone was demanded from her, and after she gave it over, the attacker then punched her so hard in the stomach that her waters broke. He only stopped from kicking her in the stomach because someone came out of a nearby house.

. . . I try not to swear on this blog . . .

The crew turned up, and took the patient to the local hospital to the maternity department.

They pre-warned the unit to meet them, as they

keep their doors locked at night.

So why, when they turned up, were the doors still locked? The excuse from the '*idiot*' midwife?

'I forgot to tell anyone'.

Followed by:

'We haven't got any beds'.

It's not bad enough that some scumbag deliberately attacked a pregnant woman, but then the people who are supposed to help her don't seem to give a damn.

The crew involved have put in a report about it, as this isn't the first time this has happened. Sometimes it seems that we are the only people doing our job properly.

Quite rightly the crew are spitting mad about the whole thing and are determined to do something about it.

I later found out from the crew that the patient later gave birth to a healthy child. Thankfully, a happy ending.

🚑 OVERTURNED

'Can you pop along to Westferry Road', asks Control, 'the fire brigade have reported an overturned car'.

'Of course', I replied, thinking there would be something interesting to blog about.

I raced down there, and indeed there was a car on its side, but the driver had run off.

Bugger.

On more than one occasion I've gone to a car crash where I would have immobilised the patient and 'blued' them into hospital, yet the patient has run off (normally because the car turns out to be stolen, not insured, or the driver is drunk). Damn them for spoiling my fun.

🚑 A NEW DEFINITION

My last patient gives me a new definition of unconscious . . .

'refusing to move or talk after having argument with girlfriend'.

To be fair, I think there is some form of underlying psychiatric problem.

But at this time of the night, you aren't going to get a mental health assessment.

🚑 AN HOUR TO GO

I've just spent the last 50 minutes with a little old lady (93), who has been vomiting since 3 a.m. An emergency GP was called, but decided not to come, instead telling the warden of the patient's flat to dial 999 for an ambulance.

The patient was a little darling, she wasn't confused, she got around on her own and generally looked after herself, and was a real pleasure to talk to. Then I looked down her nursing notes and saw that she had just finished palliative therapy for cancer.

At 5 a.m. in the morning that'll choke me up every time.

So we sat and chatted about all manner of nonsense until an ambulance was free to take her to hospital.

Why did I have to wait so long for an ambulance? Well there was another sick person at that building, and an ambulance was required about 10 doors down the road.

Coincidence?

Once more (midwives, NHS Direct and now an emergency GP) it seems that the ambulance service are the only people who actually try to do our job these days. We, and the A&E seem to be the 'safety net' that all the other services rely on to get out of doing any actual work.

It's a quarter to six in the morning; perhaps I should stop moaning and instead start thinking about my lovely warm, comfortable bed.

Palliative care means that we are treating the symptoms, rather than the incurable disease itself. Often this means that the treatment is designed to ease the patient's pain until they die.

GET THEM WHEN THEY ARE YOUNG

A couple of nights ago I got sent on a job to a 16-year-old male. He was complaining of chest pain. That makes it a high-priority call which warrants a Fast Response Unit, and therefore my attendance.

The location was in the street, so I made my way there, and met a thin-looking boy. Throughout the night I had been waiting a long time for ambulances, so I was aware that I would have to make small talk.

A quick examination and history from the patient revealed a cough, and that this was the cause of his chest pain. I then started chatting to him and found out his real problem.

He had left his familial home some time last year, and was living with a friend of the family. Then, two nights ago, he had been thrown out of that house. Too scared to go back to his mother and father, he was sleeping rough.

Skin and bone, with rotten teeth and poor skin, he had obviously been neglecting himself even before he was made homeless. I asked him about his diet, and he told me that it was junk food and a vitamin tablet. I suspect that he was living on cola and cigarettes, if not something stronger.

All while I was talking to him, he was polite, pleasant and respectful—something I don't often get from people his age.

He told me how he had fallen in with the wrong sort of people, and I realised that his chest pain was a call for help.

I decided that we needn't wait for the ambulance, and so loaded him into the car (Shhh . . . don't tell anyone, I'm not really supposed to do it), cancelled the ambulance and took him to the local hospital.

There are two types of nurses in the local hospital: those I trust to do the right thing, and those who seem to be marking the days until they can get out of there.

So I spoke to one of the nurses I trust; I told her all that I've just written and we both agreed that there was a serious need for some social services input. Thankfully, the department didn't seem too busy, so I was happy that he wouldn't get forgotten. She is also the sort of nurse who will quite happily annoy the social services until they do something.

On the way out, the young man shook my hand and thanked me.

I don't often get thanked, especially by teenagers.

Sure, he didn't need an ambulance for his physical problems. His chest pain was nothing, and while he had a poor diet, it wasn't a medical emergency, but what he did need was access to people who would care for him, and would get him on the first steps of something that I hope will lead him away from trouble.

I go to a hell of a lot of alcoholics and drug addicts, they tend to start when they are young; cruising the streets I see the men and women in their 30s who are spending the day drinking cheap cider, sitting on street corners and collecting their dole. It upsets me because they are ruining their lives.

I'm kind of hoping that we have managed to 'catch' this kid before he becomes one of them, and then becomes yet another of our 'regulars'.

Here's hoping.

NOT BREATHING

The call was to someone who was not breathing.

I threw myself into the car—a quick look at the address, and I knew where I was going. I knew the best route, I knew how to avoid the worst of the traffic and I knew I could make good time.

If she wasn't breathing, then my speed could save her life.

Blue lights were turned on, car was put into 'sport' mode (for better acceleration), trip counter zeroed and seatbelt fastened; I was ready to go.

I pulled out of the station; a quick look left and

right, then left again—no traffic. A couple of kids were standing outside the chicken shop on the corner—none of them were standing in the road (for once) so I made the sharp turn onto the road.

The first junction. Traffic here is forced into a single line, and drivers often don't see the blue lights as they concentrate on not hitting the parked cars. Thankfully, there was no-one else on the road, so I turn right and accelerate away.

The first hazard is the humpback bridge—visibility is poor, and while there is a crossing on top, kids sometimes cross just under the brow of the hill. The car hugs the road, which means that I can't see over the bridge until I'm already on top of it.

I ease off the accelerator, all clear—I gun the engine.

. . . 20, 30, 40 m.p.h. I can see the next hazard, some shops leading up to the traffic lights at the junction. I slow down, right foot covering the brake pedal. A quick check, no-one is looking to cross the road, the car heading towards me has pulled over, and I have a free run to the junction . . .

. . . and the red lights.

The siren goes on; it's loud, but the closed windows take away some of the sound. Light braking as I approach the junction; there is a queue of cars waiting for the lights (there always is) so I decide to take the wrong side of the road. I'm braking some more; it's a wide junction, so I can see what the other cars are doing. They are all waiting at the lights—the way is clear.

I swing the wheel round into a tight left turn, my folder and my bag shift in the passenger seat. The equipment in the back slides slightly, but are held in place by safety straps.

A good clear road, long and wide, just how I like them. I keep the siren going. It's sunny, and people might not see the lights. I pass the police station and a copper waves as he gets into his car. I wave back.

My eyes defocus, I don't know what I'm looking at, I try to take in the whole of the road and the pavement at once. Two kids on the right side of the road, but they are walking along, unlikely to interfere with me, one looks around at the sound of the siren.

A car ahead pulls out in front of me—Can he not see me? He pulls over and lets me past as soon as he clears his turning. No matter, I had to bleed off some speed because I didn't know if he would pull out completely in front of me.

A slight hill. Visibility is less of a problem here, but I still can't go as fast as I'd like. I clear the hill—nothing—the road is clear and I power down towards the next junction.

More shops, more cars; the lights are with me, but I know this junction well—cars will often 'jump' the lights, so again, I'm forced to slow down.

I change the sound of the siren, it becomes more insistent, shriller. My eyes are still unfocused. I note the hazards: the woman with the pram looking to cross the road, the bus in front of me looking to pull away from the bus stop, the car waiting to turn right at the junction, the bike rider (is he weaving around a bit?).

Once more, my foot covers the brake, nothing changes, the woman waits on the kerb (good girl), the bus sits there (thanks mate), the car moves over slightly, clearing my way (good boy), the bike rider straightens up (excellent).

I'm through the junction, but the traffic gets heavier, I need people to pull over and let me pass. I have a choice: I can go down the bus lane—it's clear—but people can get confused and can pull in front of me. My other option, and the one I choose in a heartbeat, is the middle of the road, forcing those on my side to pull into the bus lane, and those who can see me oncoming to pull over a little to let me pass.

I hear Obi-Wan Kenobi tell me to 'Use the Force'.

I go wide, trying to make myself as big and noticeable as possible. Lights and sirens, yellow and green livery—I should be easy to see. Some people don't pull over, I *make* them pull over. Oncoming traffic gets out of my way, they can see me from all the way down the road. One man, however, thinks it clever to flash his headlights at me and try to play 'chicken'. Obviously I don't realise I'm driving down *his* side of the road.

I swear. I swear at him loudly—he can't hear me, but it makes me feel better.

He is making me slow down. He gets out of the way, he has no choice—I give him no choice.

I continue down the road and gradually pick up speed as the traffic gets lighter. I'm constantly looking to see if any silly pedestrian wants to run out in front of me. If people weren't so daft I could drive faster.

Now for the problem road. I swing into the High Street; traffic is extremely heavy, shoppers are crossing the road. There is barely room for two lines of traffic, let alone that magical third lane I need.

I change the siren, then change it again, then

again. It's a strange sound, and it gets everyone's attention. Cars slowly try to get out of the way, a bus holds its distance. Someone decides that they can run across the road before I reach them. They are wrong, I have to jump on the brake—luckily I'm not going too fast. I swear some more, then start off again. My speed is slow; my driving has gone from speed to squeezing through gaps.

Don't look at the cars or you'll hit them I think to myself. I concentrate on the gaps between cars, some are very small. On an instinctive level I know which gaps I can make, and which ones I need to sit behind the cars, lights flashing, sirens blaring, until they make the gap wider.

How did I get here? I'm turning into the street I need—it's one way and the way ahead is clear. I'm glad, once more the parked cars make it barely wide enough for a single car.

I'm counting the door numbers—I'm looking for number 112. Odd numbers on the left, evens on the right . . .

. . . 288 . . . I speed up then slam on the brakes for a speed hump.

Again, again, again. I curse the people who think speed humps are a good idea . . .

. . . 186 . . . more humps—I pray no children are hiding between the cars . . .

. . . 172, 162, 128 . . .

I slow down. I'm trying to see the numbers, but some are small, and some are missing; while I'm doing this I'm trying not to drive into a parked car . . .

. . . 112 . . .

The door is open.

I stop. There is nowhere to park, so I'm blocking

216

the road; it can't be helped.

I grab my bags and run into the house.

'Where is she', I ask. My eyes are taking in the house, is there anyone lying on the floor?

'It's me', comes the reply.

I breathe a sign of relief.

'I've had a cough for the past week and it hasn't gone yet', she tells me.

Another normal job for me then.

Not reflective of any one job, more a reflection on all my jobs.

KNIFE TIME (WELL, ACTUALLY A SWORD, BUT YOU KNOW WHAT I MEAN ...)

This is one of a series of posts I wrote one week about the scourge of knives being used for violence.

I tend to walk the mean streets of London alone and unbothered by the thoughts of being attacked—I know that most violence is committed by people who know each other, and that truly random violence is rarer than most people think.

It was nearly three in the morning, we had all been busy that shift, so Control asked if I could attend an 'amber' call because there were no ambulances to send. I'm only supposed to go to the highest-priority 'red' calls but, to be honest, it doesn't bother me if they send me to a little old lady who has scraped her knee, and this particular job sounded fairly interesting.

It only took me a minute to find the minicab office, it is only 300 yards away from the ambulance station; it was surrounded by police cars. None of the police looked particularly panicked, so I realised that my patients probably were not seriously hurt.

The story I got was this . . .

At 1 a.m., patient one got a phone call to talk to his friend, the manager of the minicab office. Patient one collected his friend, patient two (who has only been in the country from Pakistan for a few months) and they both went to the minicab office. At the office, they were met by the manager and four other people. They were then pistol whipped, and a sword was poked into them. They were tied up and robbed of their mobile phones and £400 that one of the men was carrying. Injuries were minor, and it took them a little time to escape and call for help.

I quickly assessed both patients, and although they had been knocked around a bit, all their injuries were fairly minor, and as they were giving their statements to the police the Sergeant turned up.

(*At least I think he was a sergeant, he had some stripes on his shoulders.*)

He immediately voiced the thoughts that we were all having, that there was something 'dodgy' going on. Why would you go to a cab office for a chat at one in the morning? Why would you be carrying £400 at one in the morning to a cab office? Why were my patients being reluctant to give too many details to the police? Why would four people who you know want to torture you?

The Sergeant was polite, but firm with the men, even when they were being evasive with their answers. I was particularly impressed when he told both the men to stop talking to each other in their native language every time he asked them a question. It's a brave man who does that today, and doesn't worry about being called racist.

I left the patients with the police—their injuries were such that the FME could deal with them, and I suspect that the police would be happy to have the patients in their presence for a while.

While these people were 'victims', it's likely that the attack wasn't random in the truest sense of the word, although the use of a pistol and a sword is unfortunately getting more and more common.

KNIFE TIME II

I got sent to 'Male, stabbed in street, police present'. Luckily, I was pretty close, so I got there in 3 minutes. Lying in the street was a young male who was bleeding from the stomach.

Why?

Well, he'd run out of a shop to stop a traffic warden from putting a ticket on his car and bumped into someone, who had then pulled a knife and slashed him.

There were loads of police on scene, they'd put a dressing on him but it was soaking through with blood. I examined the wound to be sure that it wasn't a stab, and seeing that the wound wasn't that serious I cancelled the HEMS helicopter.

He refused to stop bleeding, so I spent most of my time on scene pressing on his belly with a dressing trying to stop the bleeding. It did stop eventually, and I had plenty of time to stay on scene and 'play' as the nearest ambulance was in Dagenham . . .

. . . It took *40 minutes* for the ambulance to turn

up—not their fault, and to be fair it is to be expected because we have been so busy, and undermanned.

The one good thing about the job is that it is sunny today. While I had those 40 minutes kneeling in the street, pressing on a bleeding abdomen I was simultaneously working on my suntan.

You have to look on the bright side of these jobs. Thankfully, the patient was fine. There was a bystander who was convinced that the reason the ambulance was taking so long was because the patient was black. Racism would explain the FRU and 20 police at the scene of course . . .

🚑 KNIFE TIME III

'Male, cut to arm, threatening to slice up neighbour, known psychiatric patient, wants London Fire Brigade for fun'.

That is how the job came down the computer terminal to me. Now, normally I'm not too bothered about going into potentially dangerous situations (I can run really fast if someone is chasing me), but this job rang warning bells.

(1) He has a cut to his arm; did he do it himself? If he did do it himself, then he'll probably still have the knife.

(2) Why does he want to 'slice up' his neighbour? Is he angry with them? Neighbour arguments tend to be rather nasty.

(3) What is his psychiatric history? Does he have a history of violence? Does he have a pathological hatred of the colour green? (*Our uniforms are green . . .*)

220

I decided that for this job I would wait for the police to arrive.

So, I'm sitting in my car around the corner; there is an ambulance with me and we are waiting for the police to come and protect us.

My mind starts to wander. How bad is the cut to his arm? He could be lying on the floor bleeding to death if an artery has been cut. What about the neighbour? In the time I'm waiting, has he stabbed them? When I finally go around there, will I come across a bloodbath?

I consider having a look myself. I have a stabproof vest, but my arms, legs and head are still vulnerable to having 8 inches of sharp metal shoved into them. If I did go around and get stabbed there are two things that would happen:

(1) I wouldn't get any attention until after the police turned up.

(2) I also wouldn't get any sympathy from work as they've already told me not to go near the place.

So we sit there, members of the public stare at us, and I try to chill out by listening to the latest Coldplay album (*verdict: rather good actually*).

Why haven't the fire service turned up yet? He did ask for them, and I'm sure they, like us, can't refuse a call.

They never turned up though.

The police turn up. We go around to the address and the patient is as nice as they come. He'd been (allegedly) pushed over by the neighbour and had a graze to his arm.

So, while I could have completed the job in minutes, to do so *safely* took a lot longer.

This is the sort of thing we have to think about as we go to each and every job . . . and that's just sad.

The confusion came from the patient himself as he had some mental health problems. Yet another case for being careful how you talk to our Control when you call us up.

🚐 FLAT

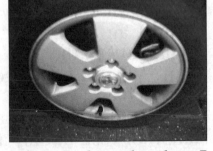

This time it isn't my fault. It was a slow leak, rather than me mounting the kerb a bit too vigorously.

I heard a 'flapflapflap' sound coming from the car, but I thought that I needed something to eat first. So I pulled up outside McDonalds and two community police officers pointed out the flat tyre.

The plan is that we are supposed to wait around until the RAC (Royal Automobile Club) come out and change the tyre. Unfortunately, they would be between 3 and 4 hours in coming.

So I got my hands dirty and changed the tyre myself. If you were in the Stratford area this morning you may have seen me scrabbling around on the floor trying to work out how to use the car jack.

I changed the tyre, but I don't trust my hand-tightened nuts to hold together when I screech round corners. So I am now sitting on station while our fitters change and check the tyre.

For some reason the phrase 'I need to get my hand-tightened nuts checked' made the woman in Control laugh.

What little I can remember about my father is that he was/is a tyre fitter—so maybe it's in the blood?

It started off as 'hit with a broomstick', but ended up resembling a cross between a riot and a carnival.

In a small road, perhaps 20 households, down on the Isle of Dogs, a family feud had finally spilled over into violence: one woman had been hit with a plastic broom, another had hurt her leg and a 10-year-old child had brandished a knife.

One of the injured parties had knocked on every front door in sight looking for witnesses, so there were around 50 people (mainly children) milling around. It was a beautiful day and people were enjoying the spectacle in the afternoon sun. Children were running around, ice creams were being sold, and teenagers were staring at the scene, smoking, snogging, and getting in the way.

The police had come in a van, and no-one was listening to what they said. They couldn't arrest the 10 year old: there were no witnesses, the child was under-age and, yes, if he **had** stabbed someone then they could arrest him.

There were half a dozen languages being spoken, and people were angry that the police and I aren't fluent in Urdu, Hindi, Somali, Turkish and Twi. They didn't realise that running up to a policeman, waving their hands around and shouting what sounded to me like gibberish, when there is someone who can translate standing next to you isn't the best way to go about things.

'She hit me', 'All three of them hit me', 'I was kicked', 'I have a broken leg' (*No . . . you don't*), 'My mum is going to have a heart attack', 'I want them arrested', 'I want this written down', 'It's been going on for ages, why haven't you done something?',

223

'Why are we waiting so long for the ambulance?', 'What are you going to do about them?', 'My mother has fainted', 'My leg is still broken'.

I suggested that the police get the riot squad down. A good idea, but they were all on day-release having a picnic.

The police were starting to lose their temper; no-one was listening and no-one cared for what the police could or couldn't do, they just wanted the attackers punished, locked up, or evicted.

People started to filter away when they realised that no-one was going to get handcuffed and thrown in the police van.

I finally managed to get to one of the 'patients'. Her family were pouring water over her head. There is a section of our community that believes that water being poured over the afflicted area will help, so I get sent to people with difficulty in breathing and chest pains who are being soaked with flannels or are dripping wet.

I'm used to strange beliefs, my mother thinks inanimate objects have feelings . . .

The water was running clear from her head, no blood. No loss of consciousness either. Looking at the 'broomstick', a light plastic pole, I'd be surprised if it even left a bruise.

The ambulances came—crews looking confused as I gave them the shortest version of the respective stories I could come up with.

The other 'patient' was complaining of a broken leg. She was still convinced she had a broken leg as she climbed up the steps into the ambulance.

Two patients, two different hospitals (we like to keep people separated in cases like this) and half a dozen police officers.

Slowly the street returned to normal and I settled down next to the Thames to do double the normal paperwork.

'No obvious serious injury'.

🚑 APOLOGIES TO ALL POLICE

Medical stuff is easy, I know exactly what to do when someone is having a heart attack, has a broken leg, or has driven their car at speed into a wall.

It's the 'social' stuff that is really tricky.

Its 3 a.m. in the morning, and I find myself going to a call, 'Female, fell down stairs'. On arriving outside the flats I heard two people arguing, and initially the female wouldn't let me into the flat. Then, a young-looking boy (he looked and sounded about 13 to me), buzzed me into the flat.

The patient had a black eye and a possible broken nose. She was covered in blood and was extremely upset.

She also refused to go to hospital, because she had her young daughter asleep upstairs.

The patient maintained that she had been out drinking, while the young-looking lad had been looking after her daughter—she didn't want to go to hospital because she didn't want to leave her daughter with the lad anymore.

I confronted her over being happy leaving her daughter to go drinking, but not to go to the hospital—she was still determined not to go to hospital.

I also asked her if she was telling the truth, and that she hadn't been assaulted. She stuck to her story that she had simply fallen down the stairs.

Unfortunately, I can't drag people off to hospital, and even if I could, I'd have to arrange care for the young daughter.

I asked the young man how old he was, and he told me he was 22.

If he is 22 then he has some serious hormone imbalance problems, as his voice hadn't broken.

So, I had a woman who looked to me as if she had been punched, refusing to go to hospital. I had a 13-year-old boy (or thereabouts) looking after her and her daughter . . . and I had heard them both arguing loudly from the street about something.

I couldn't just leave them like that, but what to do?

At 3 a.m., there is only really one thing to do, although I hated doing it . . .

. . . Call the police.

Contacting Social Services would have taken weeks to sort out the problem, and there was nothing us ambulance folk could do, so that left the police.

I know that they are busy, I know that they don't like attending this sort of thing, and I know that their hands are tied as much as mine. But I lived in hope that they could do something about this situation—at the very least get it calmed down.

I'm still not 100% sure that I did the right thing, but compared with ignoring the problem I think that getting the police involved is 'the path of least evil'.

For all I know they have a huge file on this woman.

So, to all the police who read this blog—Sorry.

226

This post is completely egotistical—but sod it, I can blow my own trumpet sometimes . . .

I think I just saved someone's life, but only because I'm honest.

It was 6:20 a.m., and I had 10 minutes to go until the end of the shift. I'd just finished a Matern-a-taxi at the other end of my patch, so I considered sitting there for the 10 minutes of my shift before 'greening up'. That way I wouldn't get another job; I could get back to station near enough in time, and by extension be safe and warm in bed before 7 a.m.

'Sod it', I thought, 'what are the chances of me getting a job in these 10 minutes'. So I 'greened up', and started heading back to station.

6:28 a.m. My computer display started buzzing, '58-year-old Male, swollen tongue'.

'Bugger'.

It's at the other end of my area, on go the lights, on goes the siren, and I key the mike to ask Control if there is anyone nearer, or anyone that finishes at 7 a.m. who could take the job. There isn't.

The problem with getting a job at 6:30 a.m. is that pretty much every other ambulance and FRU in the area finishes their shift at 7 a.m. So if they have all been on jobs, they'll sit out the last 20 minutes of the shift at hospital. Or they could all be genuinely busy.

If Control are holding a job, then they'll broadcast it over the radio and hope that someone will take it, which, to be honest, someone normally does.

So I race around there, getting there in 9 minutes. Damn, the job is a failure . . . I need to get to every job in under 8 minutes.

227

The patient has a swollen tongue alright, so much so it's nearly falling out of his head. Apparently it started swelling up from last night, and has just been getting worse.

It looks to me that he is suffering an allergic reaction, quite a serious one at that, although he has no idea what he might be allergic to.

OK, I think, if it's taken that long he has plenty of breathing time; we can wait for the ambulance, and the hospital can treat him with the nice drugs. The only drug I have in this situation is adrenaline, which can have some fairly nasty side-effects (nothing serious, just it's not a pleasant drug to have injected into you).

So we wait, have a bit of a chat, and I manage to calm him down.

'It's still getting bigger', he says. So I have a look, and it is indeed getting to a dangerously large size. If it swells much more his airway will obstruct and he won't be able to breathe.

'Alright then', I say, 'Time for that injection I told you about' . . .

. . . 500 mcg of adrenaline, straight in the muscle.

. . . 4 minutes later, and he tells me that 'It's getting smaller'.

. . . 10 minutes later and it is noticeably smaller, and he is able to talk in a much more normal voice.

His mum, 86 years old, and dressed in a little checked work pinny, comes down and offers a cup of tea.

Fifty minutes after arriving on scene, and after having a good chat about the state of English rugby, the weather and the good the NHS does, an ambulance rolls up outside.

The ambulance has also 'greened up' with 10

228

minutes to go on the end of their shift. Bless them.

I get back to station and finish my paperwork—it's now 8 a.m., one and a half hours' overtime then. Back in 10 hours to do the same again.

Then I start thinking . . . If I hadn't been honest, then I wouldn't have gotten the job, the patient's tongue would have swollen, and he could have choked to death.

All those little random decisions came together to help this patient . . .

. . . and I managed to go home with a warm glow inside, rather than the sickness of fatigue, and the dejection of yet another drunk/assault/drunken assault.

MULTIPLE EXPLOSIONS IN LONDON —JULY 7, 2005

There are a number of dead bodies from the bus bomb being stored in the BMA (British Medical Association) building. There is blood up the windows. This comes from a friend who was there when the bomb went off.

TODAY—JULY 7, 2005

A bit 'stream of consciousness' I'm afraid.

I found out about the terrorist bombs in London only because I was told by an electrician who was fitting some new wall sockets in my new flat. I rushed to plug in my small television, and found out about the bombs.

I phoned up our resource centre, as I was on my

229

day off, and they told me that I should come in and go to Newham station.

I then covered the Newham area along with others who had volunteered to come in and cover for the ambulances that were dealing with the aftermath of the attacks.

I think we had a lot less calls than we normally have; I was sitting on station for longer than normal until I, and another, manned an ambulance and took a Matern-a-taxi to an Essex maternity department.

Once the shock had settled, I started to feel immense pride that the LAS, the other emergency services, the hospitals, and all the other support groups and organisations were all doing such an excellent job. To my eyes it seemed that the Major Incident planning was going smoothly, turning chaos into order.

What you need to remember is that this wasn't a major incident, but instead *four* major incidents, all happening at once.

I think everyone involved, from the experts, to the members of public who helped each other, should feel pride that they performed so well in this crisis.

London will not be beaten, we spent 20 years under the shadow of the IRA, and are used to terrorists.

The medical staff at the BMA building did their best to save their 'civilian' staff from looking at the carnage that was left from the bomb on the bus.

The mobile phone networks appeared to be shut down—a good plan for potentially stopping more bombs from being triggered, but bad if you are trying to get into contact with relatives.

My brother considers himself very lucky: yesterday he took 40 schoolchildren to the science museum—right through the affected area.

I'm back to 'normal' work tomorrow, I wonder what it'll be like.

It took a year before the police admitted to closing down the mobile phone network. Even now I hear stories about the blasts that contradict what eyewitnesses were telling me during and just after the attack. It's strange to be 'inside' such an important story, and yet still want to write about it.

NORMALITY—JULY 8, 2005

It seems that the LAS is back to normal. No hospitals are closed, the Underground is recovering and the buses are pretty much back to normal.

London isn't in fear, and we don't seem to be hanging Muslims from lamposts. Instead, we are dealing with it and getting back to normal. This shows the resilience of Londoners no matter the faith, ethnicity or class.

I think Mayor Livingstone summed it up best when he said,

'I want to say one thing: This was not a terrorist attack against the mighty or the powerful, it is not aimed at presidents or prime ministers, it was aimed at ordinary working-class Londoners. That isn't an ideology, it isn't even a perverted faith, it's mass murder. We know what the objective is. They seek to divide London.'

Now it is up to the nurses, physiotherapists, radiographers, medical applications, therapists and

231

all the other allied services to take over the long-term and continuing healing process. These people are often forgotten but have a vital role in saving life and function.

Once more the blogsphere provided up-to-date news as well as reporting on what the mainstream media was saying.

We have a *highly* unofficial message board, there have been a lot of messages of support. Here are a few excerpts (all unedited).

The LAS and its sister services did a stupendous job today. I doubt if any city in the world could have mounted a similar response. The press talk about heroism. I'd rather talk about professionalism, organisation and effectiveness.

The street level emergency may have wound down, but a lot of our healthcare friends and colleagues are still working hard to save the lives and assure the recovery of the many victims.

I was involved in the incidents from start to finish and can honestly say no matter how much we moan and whine, it all 'came together today, be it the LAS, the LFB, the Voluntary services, hospitals, the DSOs and AOM's we slag off, the Met', the MOD plod, BTP, private amb services helped out, Miat teams, medical teams, HEMS, London buses who conveyed walking wounded, the GPs and district nurses who set up treatement centres in schools, Joe Public who gave out food to 999 personnel, the outer county services who responded to assist and anyone else I may have missed.

I might regret this, but I can actually say I was proud to work for the LAS today I've been on duty all day out in the 'burbs in south London. We've been listening in on channel 9 most of the time. To those involved you have my total admiration for a job superbly done, you're all a credit to this service.

I have to say I have never seen a service as organised as the LAS were today. I offered to go to work and when I arrived there was absolute calm and professionalism amongst every rank.

To be honest I thought it would be a nightmare but I was proved wrong. How well everyone did was astounding and a credit to the service.

Well done all involved and especially well done to all in CAC and gold control for organising what can only be described as a massive operation.

Also, well done for all the Tech, paras, ECPs and TQATs. You can feel very proud, all of you.

Thanks also to all the outer counties that assisted. Cheers Boys and girls. Your efforts will not be forgotten.

Just got home. It was a bit of a bugger out there today.

Drink. Shower. Drink. Sleep.

Talk to you all later . . .

Well done folks—went as well as could be expected.

Well done all those who attended today, and well done to CAC on channel 9.

Was listening in, and communication was second to none. Fantastic job.

Phone link went down to one of the receiving hospitals, CAC put out GB for any crew at hospital to relay blue call info. Fantastic.

I am proud today for the Service I work for.

We all moan, we have gripes about what now seem trivial matters.

Many of us came together for what was a horrendous and cowardly act of lunacy. Everyone deserves a large pat on the back safe in the knowledge you all did a fantastic job.

The thing that has annoyed us ambulance staff is that various awards have been handed out, but none of them found their way to the road-crews first on scene, or to the dispatcher(s) in Control who did an excellent job and held it all together.

🚑 HOW TO GET GASSED

You may be amused to know that at the moment I am being quarantined as a potential poison gas victim. I do have a funny taste in my mouth. More when I know myself . . .

And so what is the first thing I do? Start composing blog posts using my mobile phone. Do I have strange priorities? This post was a day after the London bombings, so people were a little nervous.

☕ CONTAMINATED

Later that day, after I'd been given the all clear I gave the reason why I was quarantined . . .

I finish a job, and start to roll back to station for a nice relaxing cup of tea. As I pass one of the roads on my route I see a *lot* of firefighters, loads of police and a Duty Officer's car.

'Hmmm', I think, 'Something interesting there'.

Then I notice a strong smell of gas.

'A-ha, that's what they are there for, someone has left the cooker on'.

So I continue on my way, with a bad taste in my mouth, and roll up to the station . . .

. . . Only to find a load of officers, strange ambulance crews (well, I say strange, but what I mean is crews from out of our sector) and some St John's people.

'Something happening?', I ask.

'Yes', says one of my friends, 'We are roaming London ready to deal with anything out of the usual'.

'In fact', she continues, 'We are here because there might be a chemical incident in Lucas Avenue'.

'Oh bugger', I think.

So I let them know that I drove past it, and they tell me to sit in my car so that I don't contaminate anyone. Apparently, one of the tests for nasty chemical stuff came back positive.

I'm not too worried, if it was anything that nasty I'd already be dead.

They retest their samples, and it's negative. The team are stood down, and I'm allowed out of the car and back to work.

Still it's nice to know that our people are still on the ball.

8:30

8:30 this morning. I'm trying to explain something to an (understandably) hysterical woman, and her two children (4 and 7 years old).

I'm trying to explain that her 37-year-old husband, and their father, is dead, and that there is nothing I can do for him.

There is nothing I can do to stop her crying. The children are in disbelief and I don't know what to say to them either.

Sometimes this job is really shitty.
Sometimes it makes you feel really shitty when you can't help someone.

STREET RESUS

My last call for yesterday was to a '65-year-old female, fall in street, possible head injury', I was only 2 minutes away, and I was happy to do a nice simple job.

Falls in the street are often minor injuries, where I have to do little other than minor treatments, and give a bit of the old Reynolds chat.

I pulled up on scene and saw a crowd of people standing around, looking fairly relaxed, and in the middle of them a woman lying on the floor. Someone was stroking her hand.

I walked up, looked down at my patient and said, 'Hello, what seems to be the problem'.

There was no answer, and her eyes kept staring ahead.

I checked her pulse, she didn't have one, nor was she breathing.

'Oh . . . bollocks', I thought.

I quickly started our treatment for this condition. Connecting my defibrillator to her (a box that monitors heart rhythm and can 'shock' the heart), I saw that she was in 'VF'. This is what is called a 'shockable rhythm', which means that I can give her heart an electric shock in an effort to restart her pulse.

When you see doctors on the telly shouting 'clear!' and then the patient's body jumping, this is what is happening.

236

So I 'shocked' her three times; when I wasn't shocking her, I was doing CPR (pushing on her chest to keep the blood flowing to her vital organs) and breathing for her with my Ambu-bag. I had to cut her clothes off (so I could attach the pads through which to deliver these shocks to her chest).

All the time I was fully aware of the crowd around me, and I was hoping that none of them had a cameraphone. None of the bystanders had seen anything, and none of them knew the woman (it looked to me as if she was just popping down the local shops).

The crowd were thankfully no trouble; actually they tried to be helpful—one person offered to help me with her breathing (I refused, because in reality it's tricker than it looks). There was another person who helped me, by running into their house and getting me some paper towels.

Why paper towels?

Well, I tend not to wear gloves, and while trying to resuscitate her, the patient had vomited up her last meal. So my hands were covered in her vomit. The paper towels were so I could wipe my hands before belatedly putting some gloves on.

So the crowd were, as we say in this part of London, 'as good as gold'. They didn't get in the way, they didn't annoy me by asking awkward questions while I was busy, and even the little kids who were watching were well behaved.

It took a long 9 minutes for the ambulance to arrive, it's not their fault, they were a long way away, and the traffic at that time of the day is pretty heavy.

We continued to attempt resuscitation, and at

two points we managed to restore the patient's pulse. Unfortunately, she later died in hospital.

Once more I was left thinking about the relatives, who would be sitting indoors wondering why mum/gran was taking so long to get back from the shops.

Also, a resuscitation attempt is not the most dignified thing to have happen to you. That this woman had to have me cutting her clothes off, me jumping up and down on her chest and her vomiting over herself, all in full view of the crowd, is not the best way in which to leave this world.

I'm hoping I have nothing but minor calls today . . .

The family wrote to the ambulance service to find out what had happened to their mother. Thankfully, I'd written everything down in a detailed fashion that day, so it was fairly easy to give them a full reply.

THINGS TO DO WHEN HIT BY A CAR . . .

Or . . . 'The reason why Barking road will be closed for an hour or two'

(1) If you have broken your arm and leg, please don't wave them around, as the sight of your bones trying to protrude through the skin is not a pretty one.

(2) If the nice ambulance man puts your neck in a hard C-spine collar and tells you to stop waving your head around, listen to him. Broken bones heal, broken necks can be a bit more . . . final.

(3) Do try to get hit down a side road. If you get hit in a main road, then the disruption to traffic will be a lot worse.

238

(4) If your 'friends' say that they saw everything and will be at the hospital, try to have the sort of friends who will actually turn up there, and not just think better of it then bugger off to whatever hole they crawled out from.

(5) Yes, I know your arm and leg are broken, but seriously, keep your neck still.

(6) If you don't want me to know your name that's OK. Just make sure you carry some identification in your wallet.

(7) Having a shaven head makes it really easy to spot a head injury, thanks for that.

(8) Loose clothing is really easy to cut off. Please dress appropriately.

(9) Keep . . . Your . . . Bloody . . . Head . . . Still!

Why the flippancy? Lets just say that he and his friends are 'well known' to the local police, and to the odd ambulance crew. Also, you want to know how we deal with nasty trauma? Dark humour . . .

The patient was a drug dealer—which explains why his 'friends' disappeared when the police turned up.

🚑 HANDBAGS

There is a special diagnostic procedure that us seasoned medical professionals use—'Handbag medicine'.

To the lay bystander it may seem that we are standing over the unconscious (or merely uncooperative) patient, rooting through their belongings, looking for something expensive to steal. For women this is normally a handbag, for men you will find us going through their wallet.

However, it is not true that we are seeking to

239

boost our wages (meagre though they are): instead, dear reader, we are trying to help the patient.

If the patient is unconscious then we need to get as much information as possible, and one way of doing this is to go through their possessions.

The best thing that we can find is a card that is big, bright and hard to overlook with 'I have epilepsy' written on the front (with the patient's name, date of birth and next of kin contact details written on the back).

The next best thing is often an address book/diary, it's especially helpful if the patient has filled in the front 'personal details' bit.

At a pinch we can use our detective skills with envelopes (opened and unopened), credit cards, GP slips, prescription forms (often very helpful), immigration or asylum documents (popular in this area) and (also popular in this area) court summons.

So, an East Anglian paramedic Bob Brotchie has come up with a rather good idea, given that people today (myself included) seem wedded to our mobile phones . . .

. . . ICE

You put the details of the person you would like contacted 'In Case of Emergency' into your phone under the name 'ICE'.

It's a good idea, and the drawbacks (the phone might be broken or separated from the patient) are the same drawbacks as anything that you would write on a piece of paper . . .

So, do it today!

True, if you are seriously injured enough, then we won't be rooting around your mobile phone (we'd be actually treating you), but it would help the staff in the hospital when they get a quiet moment.

There have been hoax emails going around saying that if you put ICE into your phone then you get your phone credits drained away. This is absolutely a hoax.

This has been a public service announcement.

I've only ever seen one mobile phone with ICE on it—but it was very helpful in that circumstance.

🚑 AGAIN?

Looks like it might be kicking off in London again. An FRU has been sent to Warren Street station, smoke has been seen. Decon Officer on station hasn't heard anything yet.

🚑 DECON

The Decontamination Officer has been told to get ready for a potential incident.

🚑 RAISED

Our Decontamination Officer has just been told that he has to come off the road and be ready on standby. This means that our level of threat has been raised a bit.

Could it be because they are worried that there may be a chemical component to an unexploded bomb?

Apparently there are chemical-suited people

241

going down into Warren Street station.

(*Probably just making sure that everything is 'clean'*).

No-one on station has had a 'normal' call for the past 40 minutes.

🚐 SHIFTING RESOURCES

One of our crews has been told to 'blue light' down to Headquarters in order to provide cover for the area affected.

Decontamination officer is still on standby.

Everyone here is fairly relaxed about the whole thing, but we are quite a way away from everything.

🚐 AND . . . RELAX . . .

So, it seems that there isn't anything chemical/biological to worry about—so no doubt the decontamination team are all disappointed . . .

The Police Commissioner has told all us Londoners to carry on as normal, but to avoid the affected areas.

The last I heard was that some of the team were looking at a 'white powder' incident—we get a couple of them a week, so it's unlikely to be anything serious.

Once more, most Londoners will look at what happened today, shrug their shoulders and make a cup of tea.

(*Something I'm going to do now . . .*)

The previous five posts were made 'live' during the failed bomb attacks on the tube and bus services a

242

fortnight after the first terrorist bombs. Thankfully no-one was hurt, but it did put us all on a higher state of alertness.

🚑 A MOMENT OF ZEN

Dark street.
A man who has been beaten unconscious.
I kneel down, and use my hand to steady me.
Under my palm I find two of his teeth.
Saturday night in East London.
If I were a cleverer person than I am, I'd have made this a haiku.

🚑 BIT OF A SURPRISE

I got a call at about 5:30 in the morning to a 'Collapsed female' with 'shouting in the background', not normally a problem, so I took advantage of the empty streets and raced there.

I narrowly avoided crashing into the ambulance also coming to the job from another direction, and so we both arrived at the house at the same time.

The patient was a middle-aged woman who had been drinking with her family, then had been some sort of argument and she was feigning unconsciousness.

Nothing unusual there.

Still no problem—the family, while concerned, were happy to agree that the patient was indeed 'faking it'.

I went out to my car to pick up a bit of kit, just in order to rule out anything medically wrong with the patient, and on the way back two men in a car parked outside asked me what was going on.

'Nothing serious', I replied, and went back into the building.

It was then that the sole male of the house cried out, 'Who's shouting outside my house?', and went outside.

I ignored him and we finished checking over the patient. As suspected there was nothing medically wrong with her.

Then the male came storming back into the house, grabbed two kitchen knives and ran outside again. The ambulance crew and I thought that this would be a good time to call for the police.

We sneaked out of the house, and stood by the ambulance—meanwhile the six women who had just left the house looked as if they were (a) arguing amongst themselves and (b) about to tear the men in the car to pieces.

The final result of the arguing, holding people back, pushing and shoving, and shrieking at the top of their lungs, was that the car drove off at high speed, missing me by about half a yard. Meanwhile, the argument continued between the sisters/cousins/whoever.

The police did turn up (and to their credit, turned up very quickly), and while they went about collecting statements there was various talk about samurai swords and the like being waved around (which isn't too surprising in this particular part of East London). We left the police dealing with what seemed to be some form of family feud.

Returning to station, we were all stood down by the duty station officer, so that we could fill in the relevant paperwork.

244

On reflection three things spring to mind:

(1) None of us were wearing our stab vests—and probably wouldn't have felt safe even if we had.

(2) Why, when I had my own mobile phone, my FRU phone, and my work emergency phone, did I use the household landline phone when calling the police?

(3) Finally, is it wrong to think 'With the paperwork we now need to do, this job'll see me to the end of my shift'?

The 'phone' thing was probably because my brain saw it there, and thought 'I can dial 999 on that', rather than taking longer on wondering which pocket of many my mobile phones are in. Thus, my brain was able to concentrate on the whole 'not getting stabbed' thing.

BAD JOB

This is a tricky post to write. Normally I would write something to emphasise how I feel, or to try and get my readers to understand what happened, or to highlight some point.

But I can't do that in this post.

All I can do right now is tell you what happened.

I got sent to a call near the edge of my 'patch', given to me as a '12-year-old female, collapse'. The navigation point wasn't accurate though, so while I could get into the right general area, it wasn't directing me right to the door. I got there fairly fast, because I always drive fast to my jobs, even if I suspect that the illness is a panic attack, a faint . . . or a broken fingernail.

I met up with the ambulance crew coming from

245

the other direction while I was checking my map, and talking to Control so as to get a better location on the patient. Control called back and gave me better directions and I told the ambulance crew to follow me.

The location was down a private road, which had huge, unmarked black speedbumps. I hit the first one at about 30 m.p.h., and had to check my mirror to make sure that I hadn't left important parts of my vehicle behind in the road.

The patient was lying in the road ahead of me, with her family standing around her. I parked my car next to her and got out to see what was happening.

The family were quite calm, and they told me that their daughter was travelling in the family car and told her parents that she felt unwell. They stopped, she got out, shook a bit and then fell onto the floor.

The parents had laid her into the recovery position and, while worried, were not screaming and crying.

Examining the patient, I saw there was a small bit of vomit in her mouth.

She then grunted.

I then saw that she had stopped breathing.

I am lucky that the ambulance was right behind me.

By now the medic on the ambulance was with me, and I told him that she had stopped breathing. I threw him my bag with the Ambu-bag in it (the bit of kit which we use to breathe for the patient), and while he started breathing for her, I cut off her clothes and connected our defibrillator.

She was in fine VF, which is a rhythm that is

'incompatible with life', meaning that her heart isn't pumping blood around her body. It is also a rhythm that we can 'shock' to try and bring her back.

I shocked her.

The monitor on the defibrillator showed asystole, which is where the heart isn't moving at all, but this can be 'normal' after giving a shock.

It was about now that the parents realised that their daughter was more ill than they thought. They asked us what was happening—all we could tell them was that their daughter was 'very ill'. You can't tell people that their daughter is dead while you are in the middle of the road, in case they mob you and the patient, and prevent you from doing your job.

By now I was doing CPR (pumping on her chest to keep the blood circulating), and she had vomited a large amount everywhere. Normally we care about getting vomit on our clothes, but in this case we weren't thinking of that.

By now the driver of the ambulance had gotten the trolley off the back of the ambulance, so we decided to 'load and go'—this girl needed to be in hospital as quickly as possible.

Her heart changed into fine VF again, so I shocked her another two times—once more she was in asystole.

We loaded the trolley onto the tail-lift of the ambulance—and it wouldn't lift!

We gave everything a kick (because there is sometimes a loose connection) and it still wouldn't lift, so I ran around and got the handle that we use to manually raise the lift, but then the tail-lift started up.

We got the patient, and the father, on board the ambulance; I jumped on to continue chest compressions, while the medic was trying to clear the airway and continue breathing for her.

The driver then put in a priority call to the nearest hospital, and started driving.

We sometimes drive fast in this job, but if there is one thing that will have us driving like a maniac it's for a nearly dead child.

While weaving our way through traffic at high speed I was keeping up the chest compressions while telling her father what we were doing.

It is hard to stand up in the back of a Mercedes Sprinter when weaving through traffic at high speed, and it is really hard to do so when some idiot in front of you decides to brake suddenly.

The vehicle lurched, there was swearing from our driver, and I grabbed a handrail. It was then I felt something 'go' in my wrist and hip.

We reached the hospital in one piece, and a nurse took care of the father, while we wheeled the patient into the Resus' room, where a team of specialists were waiting for us.

The good thing about the local hospital is that they let the parents watch the resuscitation attempt if they want. There is loads of research that shows that this is good for the family to let them know that everything was tried for their child.

I was in the reception area when the rest of the family arrived. I showed them to the relatives' room, and took the mother into the Resus' area where they were still trying to save the patient.

I was outside in the ambulance bay when I heard the family start crying, and I knew that they were crying because they had just been told that their

248

daughter/sister/granddaughter had died.

The ambulance crew and I had a little de-stress in the nurses' messroom, and then the crew took me back to my car.

There was a small amount of vomit and a bottle of water still on the scene.

I went back to station, filled in an injury report form, completed the rest of my paperwork, and spoke to Control and told them that I would be sick for the rest of the night, because by now my wrist and hip were really starting to hurt.

All throughout I wasn't 'feeling' anything, instead I was 'blank', and not because of 'shock'.

I think that its because, by my fourth nightshift, the ability to care about anything leaves me.

I was contacted by a duty officer, to check on me—he was one of the nicest officers I've spoken to. He wanted to make sure that I was psychologically alright (*I was*), and he told me that he would sort out the injury part with my station officers so that they would know what was happening.

I then went to bed.

This morning, while telling my mum what had happened, I started to feel sorry for the girl—so I know I'm not a monster.

Sometimes this job is really shitty. Everything went right with the resuscitation attempt, yet the patient still died. I'm left thinking that while I will continue, and will forget about this job (until the Coroner's office asks for a statement), that family may never recover.

I've left this post much how it is in my blog.

MULTIPLE TRAUMA AND FLOPPY CHILDREN

One of the 'problems' with working on the Fast Response Unit is, because you are so 'fast', you can often find yourself first, and only, responder on a job where you would much rather have a large number of ambulance crews.

I'm thinking specifically of the FRU who was the first, and only, paramedic on the scene of the recent London bombings.

I got sent on a job to one of our main roads, given as 'Car vs. bus'. I thought that it couldn't be too bad, as the speed of traffic on that stretch of road is about 4 m.p.h.

The police had already gotten the area taped off, and there was minor damage to the front of the bus.

Sitting some way away, nudged up against a shop, was a blue car. The first thing that hits me is that there is no way that an impact that does such little damage to a bus, spins a car through 180 degrees and throws it against a shop.

(*I later realised that what had probably happened, was that that the bus clipped the car—the driver then hit the accelerator and drove over the kerb, ending up ramming the shop*).

'Hi', said a friendly policewoman, 'there is a full-term pregnant adult female with a head injury, a baby that she was carrying on her lap and six other children, none of which had seatbelts on'.

'Gaa!', I mumbled.

I got on to Control, 'I'm going to need at least three ambulances'.

I went to check on the woman—she is indeed

pregnant, not wearing her seatbelt and she had 'bullseyed' [To 'bullseye' a windscreen, the head hits the glass and causes a distinctive ringed crack pattern. There is often hair left in the glass.] the windscreen. She had the world's tiniest cut to her head, and minor stomach cramps.

. . . A quick examination, and I'm happy she hasn't broken her neck, and is not actually that badly injured. There is nothing much to do with her.

A very quick look over the multitude of children standing around showed a swollen lip on one of them, but probably nothing serious.

A female police officer was holding the 18-month-old baby, 'I keep stroking his cheek and he keeps waking up and crying', she tells me.

I took a closer look . . . seems a bit pale.

He also looked a bit 'floppy'.

I stroked his cheek.

Not a flicker . . .

. . . Shit.

My salvation then came around the corner. An ambulance. A lovely big, yellow, blue flashing lights and sirens ambulance. An ambulance that can take this child away from me and into hospital where he needs to be.

The police officer and I jogged over to the ambulance and I gave the quickest handover to a crew ever. [Apart from the time my handover was a disdainful, 'the patient has a verruca' (incidentally, also the shortest triage note I ever wrote when an A&E nurse).] They took one look at the child and 'blued' it into the hospital. (I later found out that the child was faking it all, and was absolutely fine).

I then had to examine each of the kids to make sure that they were not hiding any serious injuries, which thankfully they were not. I then rechecked the mother of the toddler, explained why her child had gone to hospital without her, and tried to keep her calm. While doing this I was also trying to chat up one of the female police officers (*but she's having none of it*).

So I'm kept a bit busy.

I'm also being watched by an increasing crowd of people, who were not impressed by the power of police tape, and so wanted to wander over and offer advice. The police did a good job of shooing these people away, but it was a bit like Canute trying to hold back the sea.

Thankfully, there were no serious injuries (although if I had the kit, I'd have liked to have immobilised everyone involved), and the other ambulances soon turned up to ferry away the patients.

My paperwork consisted of one report form with 'Multiple patients' written on it, and a description of what I'd seen and done.

Then I went back to station, had a cup of tea and then got sent on a job on the edge of my patch, described as '12-year-old female, collapse' . . .

INTERNET SAVES GIRL!

I was going to moan.

I *was* going to tell you about the driver who tried to play 'chicken' with me. I would have told you about the brain-dead idiot who ran out, without looking, from behind a bus, causing me to leave 20-

252

feet long skidmarks (on the road, not in my pants). Maybe I would have mentioned the kid who thought it would be a fun thing to pretend to jump out in front of my car. All while on blue lights and sirens.

I might even have complained about the maternity department who told their patient to 'phone for an ambulance' (which she plainly didn't need).

I definitely would have told you about the two drivers who couldn't wait for 5 seconds before swearing at the ambulance crew and myself for 'blocking the road'. Didn't matter that we wanted to see if the guy lying on the pavement was dead or not. They only stopped shouting when two policemen sauntered over to them in their 'I can't believe you are that stupid' way, cultivated by long hours in Newham.

I would have moaned, but I've had two Chinese takeaways, so I am now feeling content and will therefore tell you about how the Internet saved the day.

I got called to a 12-year-old female who had collapsed in a block of flats.

Nothing particularly interesting about the actual collapse, but what was interesting was how the ambulance was called.

The patient was talking to a friend via a web cam.

Her friend saw her collapse (well . . . slide down under the view of the web cam). The friend then phoned the patient's house, where the phone was picked up by the patient's gran.

Gran then rushed into the patient's room where she saw the patient collapsed on the floor. Gran then phoned for an ambulance.

We turn up.
We save the day.
Yay for us.
So all hail the Internet, saviour of teenage girls!

SHEER BLOODY TERROR

Very little scares me: violent drunks, dark alleys, terrorist bombs, careening around corners at silly speeds—none of these things bother me. But I do have one completely irrational fear . . . and today I faced that fear.

Terror is often depicted as happening at night, in the middle of a thunderstorm, but for me terror happened on a sunny Monday morning.

The first job of the day was nice and simple, a little old lady with a leg infection who needed some antibiotics that can only be given at hospital.

Just don't ask me why this was a high-priority call, and therefore needed a Rapid Response Unit.

I spent some time chatting with the patient and her relative—nice enough folks just feeling let down by their GP. Little did I know the trauma that would soon be inflicted on me . . .

The ambulance crew turned up, and put the carry-chair next to the patient. The patient was having severe pain on standing, so one of the crew and the patient's daughter grabbed an arm each and gave her some help standing.

During this I was standing in the kitchen door, and the other crew was standing in the hallway door.

Then I saw it.

I have big hands, and the spider that ran up the back of the patient was just a shade smaller. I was

254

standing some way away and even with my poor eyesight, I could see its huge fangs, its hairy legs, and an evil glint in its eyes.

I froze.

'I'm not f**king wrestling with that monster,' was the first thing that sprang to mind.

Sprinting onto the patient's head it sat there for a moment, no doubt deciding which of us would make the tastiest meal.

The daughter screamed, the (female) crew helping the patient screamed, the (male) crew standing in the doorway swore, screamed, and ran out into the hallway to hide.

'Get it off! Get it off', the daughter screamed.

The spider decided to sit on the face of the patient, its legs gripping the patient's ears like a facehugger from the 'Alien' films.

'Eeek!' screamed the patient.

The daughter then smacked her mother right in the face, and the spider went flying across the room. I had visions of it smashing into a vase, bringing it crashing to the floor.

(*Did I mention that this spider was fairly large?*)

I stood there like a lemon, my long-dormant arachnophobia flaring into action—I was petrified.

I don't like killing ~~things~~ animals—I even rescue the silverfish from my bath before washing my hair—but if this thing came near me it would be a fight to the death.

The patient sat alone in the room in the carry-chair, breathing heavily from her daughter's assault.

Neither of the crew wanted to go near the patient in case the spider was merely lurking . . . biding its time until it could attack. My bags were taken off me and I was told in no uncertain terms that it would be me who would approach the corner in order to actually collect the patient.

A deep breath, a muttered Litany against fear, and I scooted across the room and, keeping my eyes on the many dark corners, swiftly bundled the patient up and got her out of the house.

'Don't worry', said the daughter as we left the house, 'Mum's dog will soon eat it'.

Depends how big the dog is, I thought . . .

I was left a comment on my website by the (male) crewmember who screamed like a little girl (I only refrained from screaming because I didn't want to attract its attention). He told me that he thought he heard the doorbell and was going to see who it was. This is a blatant lie.

THE BENEFITS OF LOVELY WEATHER

It's funny how the nice weather we are having at the moment makes you look at everything in a different, happier light.

Take today for example, I was sent to a 'Life status questionable' in the street. Now a 'life status questionable' is supposed to mean that the person who called us doesn't know if the person is alive or not.

What it means in reality is that the caller has either driven past in a car without stopping, or the patient has such an offensive smell that the caller dare not get close to them.

So, I rush to the scene and find an alcoholic sitting in the street. Around him are his four alcoholic friends.

256

The person who made the call is nowhere to be seen.

'He's just tired', I'm told by one of his friends.

'Why's that?' I ask.

'Well, he's just walked from Whitechapel' (Whitechapel is about 6 miles away).

'Oh', I say, 'No wonder he is having a bit of a sit down'.

'This'll help him out', says one of his friends giving him a can of Special Brew.

The ambulance crew turn up, and we all have a little chat on the corner of the street; everyone is as nice as pie, and no-one is really injured.

I know that I should be annoyed (waste of ambulance time and resources, waste of lives on the part of our alcoholic friends), but it wasn't really their fault that an ambulance was called.

And the sunny weather just put everyone in a nice mood.

Long may it last . . .

Of course, saying that, nice weather means that young men drink long into the night, and then beat each other up.

The counter to this is that when the nights are long and the days are short and dark I find myself stomping around in a foul mood. I'm very fickle.

☕ WAITROSE

Good karma is due for the duty manager of Waitrose who gave the ambulance crew (and, more importantly, me) some free doughnuts for helping one of their shopgirls.

Yummy.

257

🚑 SORRY

I spent an absolute age trying to get this post right. Eventually I just threw up my hands in surrender and posted it in the format below. I hated it, but a lot of my readers liked it.

Dear patient,

I'm sorry.

I know you thought that you were going to die peacefully, but we have to try and save lives, even though you were terminally ill. Your husband didn't want you to die yet, neither did your daughter.

I'm sorry that when I reached you, you were breathing your last. It meant that I had to lift you off your bed onto the hard floor.

I'm sorry that I had to do that, but it is the only way I could do effective chest compressions. I'm sorry I had to do the chest compressions; I know I broke some of your ribs, but please understand that it is a known side-effect of trying to keep your heart pumping.

I'm sorry that we had to put those needles in your veins, but you needed the fluid. You also needed the drugs that helped your heart beat, but it was probably painful.

I'm sorry that we had to pump air into your lungs; it can't have been nice for you, but we needed to keep your vital organs supplied with oxygen.

I'm sorry that because of the air in your pleural space we had to push two large needles into your chest. I don't know if you felt it, but it did help reinflate your lungs.

I'm sorry that your husband didn't quite

understand what was going on—we tried to explain, and I think that at the end he did realise that you probably weren't going to wake up.

I hope you didn't mind when we had to keep passing a couple of hundred joules through your body. It made your body jump, but it's not your fault.

I don't know if it hurts. I hope that it didn't.

I know that the journey into hospital wasn't the smoothest ride, and the sirens were loud, but we did need to get you into hospital quickly.

I did remember to wrap the blanket around you so that anyone standing outside the hospital doors wouldn't see that you were naked.

But . . .

. . . I'm *not* sorry that we, and the hospital were able to keep you alive long enough for your family to arrive and gather around you.

I hope that there was a part of you that was still aware of what was happening, and was able to hear their words of love.

I hope that it was worth the pain so that you could hear those words, and feel their presence.

When I left you at the hospital your heart was beating and you were breathing. I hope that your end was without pain.

🚑 SAVED ONE!

I know it's a rare thing, but we actually managed to save the life of someone! It was bloody hard work mind you, so I wouldn't want to do it too often . . .

I got sent on a job with very few details; all I got was 'Male, unknown age, unconscious, unknown cause'. I knew roughly where the address was so I rushed around there, and saw the ambulance pulling up at the same time.

I quickly checked my computer screen and saw that I had gotten to the location in under 8 minutes. Whatever happened now the government would consider this job a success.

There was something about the family member who let us through the security doors that set my 'spider sense' tingling. That 'something' was confirmed when the ambulance crew and myself walked into a bedroom and saw a rather dead-looking 30-year-old male lying on the lower part of a bunk bed.

I must admit that my first thought was 'I wonder how long he has been dead?', because if he had been dead for a while, we wouldn't have to attempt a resuscitation. We quickly pulled him from the bed and laid him on the hard wooden floor.

'*Grrrooooooollll*' was the noise he made.

I'm very used to dead people making unusual noises: it's normally as a result of their last breath leaving their body.

We quickly hooked up our heart monitor and checked for a pulse.

His heart was beating!

He took a shuddering breath.

The patient wasn't breathing often enough to maintain life, so we would have to take over breathing for him, which we did using a bag and mask.

One of the crew lay on the floor and peered down his throat. Would we be able to intubate him? (intubate = stick a breathing tube down the patient's throat in order to protect their airway)

'Nope', she told me, 'his airway is too tight'.

We picked up the (heavy) patient and wheeled him out of the house and into the ambulance.

Another attempt at securing his airway . . .

'No chance', she said, 'His airway is the size of a pencil'.

This explained why I was finding it hard work to force air into his lungs.

'Perhaps it's his asthma', I suggested, 'shall we get some salbutamol into him?' (Salbutamol is an asthma medicine that is inhaled—we can use various complicated connecting tubes to give this drug while I continue to 'bag' him).

'Let's give some adrenaline as well', I said; seconds later it had been drawn up and given (giving adrenaline is another treatment for asthma).

(*Why was I the one making all the suggestions? Well the crew were busy connecting monitoring equipment, gaining intravenous access and doing other tricky things—I had the simple job of breathing for him, so I had plenty of time to think about our next step of treatment.*)

Then it was time for the run to hospital. By now the patient's chest was getting harder and harder to inflate. The levels of oxygen in his blood were lower than I would have liked, but it was pretty understandable considering how incredibly close he was to death.

His chest got so tight that it ended up with two of us 'bagging' him—I would hold the mask to his face, while one of the crew was using both hands to squeeze the breathing bag. I can still feel the pain in my arms where I was using all my strength to squeeze the bag in order to force air down his tiny

261

airway and into his spasming lungs.

Then he vomited blood—well, 'vomit' is an understatement, he actually went off like a geyser—bloody vomit flew up to the ceiling of the ambulance, on the walls, over my arms, onto my trousers and covered my face and glasses.

I have learned, however, to keep my mouth closed when this happens . . .

We got to hospital and, as we were entering the Resus' bay, the patient was starting to breathe for himself—and by the time we had cleaned up the ambulance (and my face) the patient was sitting upright and was talking.

He had made such a recovery that the staff at the hospital had trouble believing that he was as ill as we told them he had been.

(*Until they checked his blood levels, and on getting the results ended up sending him to intensive care*).

A quick round of pats on our collective backs, and it was back to work . . . where my next job was a 30-year-old with a painful foot for the past week.

🚑 A CALL TO ARMS

An attempt to show my political leanings.

It's that special time of the year again, when death-dealers descend on Newham to enjoy the 'Defence Systems and Equipment International exhibition'.

It's an arms fair.

In *Newham* of all places.

I'm always worried that the local gangs are going to storm the fair and loot it of some 'interesting' souvenirs. Then, for the next couple of months, I'll find myself dodging cruise missiles and landmines rather than the usual broken bottles, knives and dog turds . . .

Both the mayor of Newham, and the mayor of London want the exhibition to stop coming here, but it still comes, bringing with it massive disruption for the people of Newham.

So there will be lots of demonstrations (some have already taken place, such as a street party), but as the exhibition starts tomorrow we are expecting things to start warming up a bit. I haven't seen any ~~soap-dodgers~~ protesters yet, but I'm guessing that tomorrow will see the banner-wielding population of Newham increase a thousand-fold. At the moment it seems that a lot of their tactics involve blocking various roads that control entry to the exhibition.

So far I have seen a veritable army of police arriving, shields at the ready (4 000 police taken from other duties to cover the event). Obviously, this leaves the rest of London a bit short on policing. I've seen convoys of riot police making their way to the area, and this morning there appeared to be random vehicle checks. For the police it must be nice to have so much overtime available.

On our part, the LAS have manned an extra ambulance or two for the duration of the exhibition. Sitting in the sun watching people shouting seems like an easy way of getting some overtime. We are also doing other things, but it's probably not a good idea to tell the world and his wife about it. I just hope that the exhibition organisers are paying for our services, after all, it's not like they are short of money.

It might be interesting to print out a spotter's card of dictators, warlords and despots just to see how many you can catch turning up in unmarked limousines.

I must admit I'm torn. I like the police, they are always helpful; they do a job that is remarkably difficult and when I've needed help they've always turned up and been very useful.

But . . .

I really sympathise with the protesters, and if I wasn't working, then I'd probably be there amongst them waving a banner and trying not to get stood on by a police horse.

So I'll sit on the fence and say that they are both going to be a huge pain in the backside because they are both going to block roads, probably injure each other, and will cause traffic jams when I'm planning on going home.

The Philosophy of Reynolds—*'balance through the dislike of everyone'*.

MERCY! MRSA!

The media has reported a fair bit about MRSA in ambulances of late; one of my commenters has asked how the London Ambulance Service deals with patients who are MRSA positive.

(*Note: I'm also writing this to avoid losing my job by posting about a family who have called an ambulance more than seven times in the past week for the same illness.*)

Primarily the problem is that we just don't know who is MRSA positive. MRSA is prevalent in the community, and I would suggest that most nursing homes have plenty of colonised residents. I remember working in hospital, having to swab everyone coming in from a 'high-risk' environment, which meant anyone from a nursing home, or another hospital.

It takes time to swab and grow a culture (3 days if I remember correctly), and each test costs a not inconsiderable amount of money.

If a patient is MRSA positive, then our infection control booklet tells us that we should use our 'personal protective equipment' (our uniforms) plus what are known as 'universal precautions'— essentially latex gloves.

To clean an ambulance after transporting an MRSA-positive patient we use 'System 1' and 'System 2 or 3'.

System 1: Detergent.
System 2: Chlorine spray.
System 3: Alcohol.

Anything the patient has come in contact with is wiped with detergent, and then we either spray it with chlorine solution, or wipe down with alcohol wipes.

The other problem that we have is that we are so chronically overworked that we often only have a little time to clean the ambulances. If you are having a heart attack, then you won't be impressed if all the ambulances on duty are off the road waiting to dry.

When the LAS do something, we often do it right. Our boss realised that the ambulances aren't as clean as they should be, and that road staff didn't have time to 'deep clean' ambulances every shift. The solution was to contract an outside firm who now cleans and stocks our ambulances for us and from what I have seen, they do a pretty good job.

So, every night a gang of underpaid workers clean as many ambulances as possible. This 'make-ready' crew are paid a frankly pitiful £6 an hour, working from 1 a.m. to 6 a.m. They can clean around 16 ambulances a night using industrial cleaning materials. Every month they are quality controlled by random swabbing. So far they have only had good results.

So, I personally think that the LAS is doing something positive and effective against the spread of MRSA.

It will never be eradicated, unless we force everyone at gunpoint to use alcohol gel after every physical contact (and this includes 'civilians') and enforce daily antibacterial showers for the entire population of the world. However, we can do our best to prevent the spread of MRSA (and other, nastier diseases).

🚑 80/50

A strange day; it wasn't that hot, but all I seemed to be doing was going to young women that had fainted.

A *lot* of women who had fainted.

It started off on the 30th floor of a skyscraper in Docklands, which had a lovely view. People were having meetings around tables in the expensively furnished corridors, and all the office walls were made of glass . . . which made me glad that I didn't have to undress the woman who had fainted.

Then it was across the road to another woman

who had fainted in another (less well furnished) office.

Then a bit of a run north to yet another woman who had fainted.

Then a gentleman who had fainted on the bus.

Then a woman who had fainted in the local shopping centre.

It seemed like people were dropping like flies.

The *really* unusual thing was that the blood pressure of all the patients was 80/50, which is really rather low.

It also struck me as interesting that the first of my fainters was near the Arms fair, and then got progressively further and further away . . . I didn't think to check the direction of the wind . . .

Thirteen jobs today. I am, as they say, bloody tired.

🚑 UNCONSCIOUS? (TRICKS OF THE TRADE)

Some people seem to think that faking unconsciousness is a good idea: either they are mentally ill, drunk, or more commonly, have had some form of argument and have decided to 'go unconscious'.

For some reason, benefit offices and rent payment offices are popular places, as are police cells, magistrates' courts and the checkouts of supermarkets.

The easiest and quickest way to see if someone is faking unconsciousness is to lightly brush your finger against their eyelashes. If their eyes flicker, then they are almost certainly faking it. Also, if they try to keep their eyes closed when you try to open them, they are definitely faking it. Another way of checking is to hold their hand over their face, and let it drop. People tend to be reluctant to let their hand hit them on the nose, and so the hand will instead magically drop to one side.

The other giveaway is that they open their eyes to look at you when they think you aren't watching them . . .

But what happens if someone is able to wake up, yet is refusing to?

Let me quickly explain an important part of measuring someone's 'Glasgow Coma Scale'. The Glasgow Coma Scale is a way of measuring how deep someone's level of unconsciousness is. Part of this process of assessment is how they respond to pain.

The official method of applying this pain is to push hard against the upper part of the eye socket. This does no damage but is apparently painful.

. . . Not to me it isn't, and not if you are deeply drunk.

So there are other painful stimuli, one of which (my favourite) is the 'sternal rub', where you rub the knuckles of your hand against the patient's breast-bone. Some lily-livered people think that this assessment is too close to assault, but I would ask them to consider that if we didn't get drunks to wake up, we would be forced to undertake invasive medical procedures on them in order to ensure that their airway is clear. If you can tolerate my sternal rub then there is something seriously wrong with you, and you need emergency treatment—if you wake up then I have effectively 'cured' you.

Either way the assessment is complete.

Of course I did get a broken rib for my troubles when 'curing' an unconscious drunk who had sexually assaulted a female pedestrian. I also can't see how one way of causing pain may be assault, but another isn't.

The moral of this story is simple: don't pretend you are unconscious, because we will know, and don't pretend to be unconscious when you are drunk, because it can get painful for you.

My favourite tale of how to uncover a pretender in a hospital setting was a doctor, who would loudly ask for the 'brain needle', to draw off some brain fluid from the unconscious patient via the ear. Of course, he would continue, the patient needed to be unconscious because otherwise they might flinch and the needle go into the brain itself. This was normally followed by the patient 'waking up' and asking, 'Doctor, where am I?'.

REPRIEVE

Four miles away 'Bob' was about to stop breathing.

Bob's friends had seen him come out of rehab' earlier that day; they had then invited him around to their flat where they then saw him inject some heroin.

Bob's friends had then watched him pass out for half an hour, and then his breathing had slowed and he had gone a funny shade of blue.

His friends decided that now might be a good time to call for an ambulance.

I arrived at the same time as the police, who were there to make sure that I was safe.

One of the residents held open the main door to

the tower block.

'Another fucking junkie?', she asked, 'It's a fucking crack house up there'.

We got in the lift, carefully avoiding the nasty-smelling puddle in the middle of it, and I hit the button with my gloved finger.

Sure enough, if you worked in film making and were asked to create a set based on a crack house this is probably what you would come up with. Actually, as crack houses go, it wasn't too bad— there were no human faeces spread around for a start. No carpets either, which is a good thing because it's easier to spot the wet patches on lino.

To give Bob's friends some credit, they had managed to put him into the recovery position in the middle of the kitchen. Bob had either vomited, or his friends had poured some water on him. Either way there was something sticky on the floor around him.

For the second time on this job I was really glad I was wearing gloves.

His friends were both clutching cans of cheap, but strong lager. One of them was so skinny he would have made Iggy Pop look like Pavarotti. I left the police talking to them.

Bob had decided that breathing four times a minute was quite enough for him but the blue pallor of his skin, and my training, would tend to disagree with him. Bob was very nearly dead; I suspected that he would soon break the first habit of his life—the habit of breathing. I put an airway down his throat, pulled out my Ambu-bag and started breathing for him.

He soon pinked up and perked up, and his breathing got better, so I could stop 'bagging' him. I could relax a bit, and watch him while I waited for

270

the ambulance to arrive—which wasn't long.

We moved him into the carry-chair, being careful not to stab ourselves with any needles that might be lying around him (or in his clothing, his pockets, or lying underneath him). It was about now that he started to wake up.

Another life saved, although no doubt his habit will kill him one day.

It strikes me as ever so annoying that for some reason I can manage to save heroin addicts, but not 12-year-old girls.

MORE

At least three people in my area have called an ambulance because of being in the early stages of labour.

Something else that upsets/annoys me is that a family bought in their dead toddler by private car, and never thought to call an ambulance.

Make of that what you will.

I was particularly annoyed that evening. Most of my calls were to people wanting to give birth, yet were so far away from actually giving birth they could have walked to the hospital. Then I hear about the dead toddler who needed an ambulance and, because of the way they died, might still have been alive today if an ambulance had been called when they started to get sick.

SURPRISE

I walked in through the door and there she was,

271

standing stark naked in a pool of her own blood.

Heavily pregnant, she was sobbing while blood ran down her legs. Her neighbours were making an attempt at comforting her, all the while trying to clean the blood away. Meanwhile, between great sobs of tears, the patient was trying to fit a sanitary pad to herself.

As I write this I can still smell the blood.

The ambulance was 10 minutes away.

Someone in my comments box made an off-colour remark and was berated by my regular commenters. I remember this job because while the patient was black, the neighbours who helped her were two white 'granny' types. It was nice to see people being helpful across supposed cultural barriers.

WAKE-UP CALL

I walked into work at 6:15 a.m., I'd been awake since half past five. Well, I say awake—what I actually mean is that although I was somehow moving around, and managed to drive to work, my mind was still comfortably asleep in bed back home.

I start to check the equipment in my FRU; most of it is there, but I'm missing a few pieces of kit— expensive pieces of kit, probably sitting on a vehicle elsewhere in our complex.

Then my phone went off. 'Hello', said Control, 'We've got a cardiac arrest for you'.

I jumped in the car, checked the address, then saw the age of the patient . . .

. . . 42.

Control also sent a message that the patient's

wife is doing CPR. This meant that he might just have a chance of surviving this . . .

I raced towards the address; it didn't take long, although because of recent rainfall, I was sliding all over the road.

It's only when I turned onto the road that I realised that I'd been to this address before. I'd spoken to this man previously; he seemed like a decent person. I *know* him.

I ran in through the door; the hallway was clean but I could not see anyone, so I shouted out.

'Up here', came the cry of an obviously distressed woman.

'Sounds genuine', I thought.

So I bounded up two flights of stairs and into the bedroom, where I saw the wife performing pretty effective CPR on her dead husband.

She was crying.

I took over. Connecting the patient to my monitor/defibrillator I saw that the patient's cardiac rhythm was asystole—there is no activity in his heart at all.

Now came the tricky part. I was on my own, and there are a lot of things that I had to do very quickly.

I did 15 chest compressions—this would hopefully get some oxygen to his essential internal organs. But to continue doing this I needed to get his lungs full of air. So the next thing I did was is connect up the 'Ambu-bag' to my oxygen cylinder.

I tilted his head back and used the Ambu-bag to inflate his lungs twice.

I started another 15 chest compressions.

Downstairs I heard the crew entering the house.

'Top floor mate', I shouted, 'Job is as given'.

When I say the 'job is as given', I mean that it was given to us as a cardiac arrest, and that it is indeed a cardiac arrest and not a faint/panic attack/cough or belly ache.

It seemed like ages, but when I later checked the times, the crew were less than 2 minutes behind me.

Three people came bounding up the stairs. The FRU from another station had jumped into the back of the ambulance—he was waiting on station for the previous shift to return when the crew got the call.

I continued the chest compressions. One medic put a breathing tube down the patient's windpipe, the other gained access to a vein, so that we could give essential medications. The last crewmember was doing the very important (*but often underrated*) job of looking after the wife.

After about 9 minutes of this treatment, the rhythm on the heart monitor changed. It looked suspiciously like a decent heart beat.

I checked for a pulse.

I found one!

The patient then spent the next couple of minutes (while we were preparing to move him) slipping in an out of either having a pulse, or having a 'shockable rhythm', which needs an electric shock to revert this back into a heart rhythm 'compatible with life'.

He ended up getting defibrillated twice before we could load him onto the carry-chair, lug him down two flights of stairs and into the back of the ambulance.

We then found a member of the public upset that we were blocking his parking space. He was blocking the only exit that the ambulance had.

One of the crew had a word with him. She is much more polite than I would have been.

He moved out of the way rather quickly.

As there were three crew in the ambulance, they didn't need my help, so I followed behind them so that I could get my equipment back. By the time I reached the hospital the patient was being prepared for transport to the intensive care unit.

The wife gave the crew a hug, and sobbed how grateful she was. Even the doctor at the hospital complimented us on a job well done.

But, failing a miracle, the patient will die—he was without oxygen for too long.

Once more it seems that we are just making time for the relatives to say goodbye. But for us it still seems like a success.

This is the patient I mentioned earlier who was having a 'thrumming' heartbeat. It was a damn shame.

🚑 'CARE' HOME

I usually only tend to see the bad nursing homes. I'm not talking about nursing homes where the patients are abused in the traditional sense, but rather where they seem to have simply been . . . left.

I went to one the other day, run by a large prestigious private health-care company, it is clean and looks very pretty . . . but I'd rather die than spend my final days there.

The patient was 90 or more years old and had been bleeding from her vagina since 9 a.m. that morning. I was called at nearly noon. They had left her bleeding for 3 hours.

I found her lying on a towel on a plastic bed; there was no sheet and the only bedclothes she had was a single sheet across her body.

Her room was clean, but was empty of anything personal—there were no pictures, no letters, no ornaments . . . nothing.

I looked at her drug chart. She was on two types of painkiller, but for the past 5 days, those, and her other medications were marked as having been 'spat out'. I'm guessing that this was because of her advanced dementia, rather than an informed refusal.

If she was spitting out her medicines, I wonder if she was also spitting out her food and drink. There was a bottle of drink next to her bed, but there was no way that she would be able to reach it. Looking at her skin, she did look dehydrated.

The 'nurses' all walked with the speed of arthritic turtles, and I had to struggle to find one that knew anything about the previous visit the patient had made to the hospital. Actually, I struggled to find a nurse that knew much about anything.

'I don't know this drug', I said to one of the nurses testing her, 'what is it for?'

I knew what the drug was for, but the nurse didn't . . .

One of the care assistants sat on the end of the patient's bed. The patient seemed a bit distressed at this, but it was hard to tell as she was staring at the ceiling. The carer suddenly got off the bed, and this obviously caused the patient pain as she cried out.

The care assistant left the room, and I was left trying to comfort the patient, holding her hand and apologising.

I wondered what this woman had seen, what she had lived through. I could imagine her dancing in the 1930s, being married and having children (her daughter was on the way to the hospital already), raising her children while living through the war, maybe working as part of the Land Army. I thought about her husband, probably long dead, and the friends she had also probably outlived.

It always depresses me to think that some people end up in homes like this, where the care is slipshod, and her life is now just an accumulation of numerous small acts of omission.

EPILEPTIC FIT

We got called to a 'Female—epileptic fit' in the street. This was a call that was sent to us by the police. Now, I may be accused of being overly cynical, but when the police call us to an 'epileptic fit' it is normally because they are arresting someone, and in order to avoid going to the police station the person fakes a fit. There are ways and means of detecting when this is the case, some of which I have mentioned previously. Even though this was the likely explanation for this job, we still rushed down there, fully prepared for it to be genuine.

We turned up to see a car being towed away, and the police that met us had a slight smirk about them. The finely tuned sixth sense I have made me suspect that the police were hiding something from me. We were led to the patient, who was lying in a darkened alleyway, with her boyfriend standing over her.

As is my normal approach, I said something along the lines of 'Hello love, can you open your eyes for me', I brushed the thick, long hair from out of her eyes, and, being unable to see the patient properly pulled out my torch and shone it in her face. At first I thought it was just a very unattractive woman, then I brushed the hair back a bit further and that caused the wig to slip . . .

This female was born a man.

Now, I have no problem with transsexuals. I know a couple in a social situation, and apart from the time I caught one of them going to the bathroom in a pink dressing gown and pink bunny slippers, their gender doesn't pay any part in what I think of them (*as with gay men, I just think, 'Great! More women for me!', of course it doesn't work out like that, but I live in hope*).

The hardest bit is working out whether to call the patient 'he' or 'she'. So I asked the boyfriend.

It looked as if the patient had had a genuine epileptic fit, and so we got 'her' onto the ambulance and started our treatment. I managed to get a lot of the details off of her boyfriend. We got her into hospital, where we found out that she was not unknown to the hospital. By now she was starting to come around.

As she and the boyfriend didn't live in the area that we found them in, I asked what she was doing there. Apparently, she had parked the car on the estate, then someone had stolen the keys. Given what she was wearing (pink furry moon-boots, tight leather miniskirt, tight pink top, and a leather/furry frock jacket), and what I saw when I peeked at her previous medical history, I wonder if she was one of those 'ladies of the night' that we often drive past.

I mean, most of them look a bit rough, but having been born a man might explain a lot . . .

Yet another 'dinner party' story.

COMMUNITY RELATIONS

(*WARNING: It has been a while since I was in education, so I don't know the current ideas on political correctness, so if the post below is insulting, I'm sorry. You should know by now that I treat everyone the same. If you think I'm racist, then check out my archives. However, it's not against the law (yet) for me to say that I think religion is a generally silly idea*).

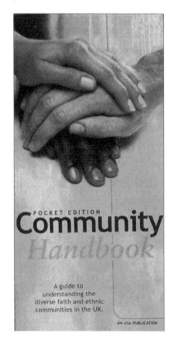

POCKET EDITION
Community
Handbook

A guide to
understanding the
diverse faith and ethnic
communities in the UK.

AN ASA PUBLICATION

Written by the Ambulance Service Association, *The Community Handbook* (pocket edition) is an easy reference guide to many of the ethnic groups that we may come across. Of course, in London there are around 200 different ethnic groups, so any 'comprehensive' handbook would weigh a ton—we get a two-page spread of some of the commoner ethnic groups in the UK.

It's very pretty, and I can imagine it possibly being useful for ambulance trusts who do not have a large 'ethnic' population. But I work in Newham, where the 'ethnics' outnumber the WASPs, and I've found that you tend to pick up on other peoples' culture pretty quickly, as in a week or two, on the job.

One amusing point of the book is that for a lot of cultures, it says that you should remove your shoes on entering the house. Yet one of the main things we were told in ambulance school was that you never take your boots off, as it's just too dangerous. I've only once been asked to remove my boots before, when I was entering a mosque. I explained that I couldn't and the head bloke there told me not to worry, as the sick person was more important (he was as well—he was having a heart attack).

For a number of cultures, the book tells us that we should speak through the head male family member. Again, in practice I've never come across this. What I do tend to come across is a 7-year-old girl doing the translating for the whole family, which is why I think you have a lot of very 'grown-up' Asian girls. Language is always a problem, but I've found that although people tell me that they can't speak English, it is more probable that they don't have the confidence to try. I always try to talk to the patient, and then the relatives will translate the odd tricky word.

Various cultures also apparently have a taboo about men dealing with women. Again, something I have very little trouble with, as I'm not about to perform gynaecological examinations on my patients. The only time I've found that it might be an issue is with delivering babies, but if there isn't a woman around then I've found that people are just plain happy that there is someone around who knows what to do.

Although, having seen some of the ethnic grannies, and their attitudes to their granddaughter having a baby (something along the lines of, 'Stop being a wimp, and push it out')—I suspect that they have more idea about delivering babies than I do.

I can't see any culture being happy about having their women undress alone in front of strange men.

The book also has little sections on 'Customs around Death'. I'd like to think that we are so successful at treating people that we don't have to deal with it that often . . .

To be honest, a lot of the book is trying to teach us to suck eggs. As long as you have some semblance of common sense, and are polite and respectful to everyone (*except maybe drunks . . .*), then you shouldn't have any problems. If in doubt, ask, is my motto and I've learned quite a bit about other cultures just by asking the patient. I'm guessing that a lot of ethnic people have come across a fair bit of unconscious culture clash, and have developed their own strategies for dealing with it.

Please note how Reynolds has made special effort to make everything positive in the above post. Note how he hasn't mentioned that some people have a huge chip on their shoulder about their culture, or how one culture seeks to emulate the worst qualities of another culture, or how a lot of non-drunken violence seems to be 'ethnic' vs. 'ethnic' violence. Just remember, I dislike everyone equally—I'm an equal opportunities cynic.

🚐 SEVEN WITNESSES

I got sent to a job 'Female 14, collapse in back of police van'. Nothing suspicious about that—we often get people collapsing when they are being arrested/evicted/given final notice/have the repossession people around.

So there they were, in a side turning just off a main road. I parked up and could tell from the relaxed attitude of the police that it was probably nothing too serious. One look at the patient confirmed this—she would have to go to hospital (to protect everyone against being sued), but she was fine. I examined her vital signs and everything seemed to be normal.

The ambulance turns up and I'm just handing over the information about the patient when a woman in an SUV turns down the (now blocked) side turning. Realising that she was not going to fit between ambulance and police van, she started to reverse.

The ambulance crew, the four police officers and myself could all see what was going to happen next.

'STOP!', shouted the policeman.

'Stop!', shouts (slightly less loud) one of the ambulance crew.

'Oh dear . . .', I whispered under my breath.

CRUNCH . . . went the (slightly battered) SUV against an absolutely pristine vintage Jaguar.

'FUCK!', went the driver of the Jaguar (quite understandably I feel).

'You *muppet*', muttered the police officer.

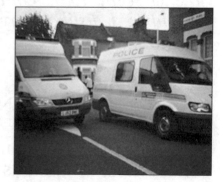

If you listened carefully you might have heard a little snigger from someone on the ambulance side of the seven witnesses of this act of 'Driving without due care and attention'.

Not from me . . . obviously.

The patient went into the back of the ambulance, and I was left chatting to one of the policemen.

'I bet', I said, 'She doesn't have any insurance . . .'

'Well', he replied, 'It seems that half the people around here seem to think it's optional'.

So, I have a little eavesdrop, and sure enough, she had no insurance. The driver tried to get angry at the police, but this soon vanished when she realised exactly how much trouble she was in.

(*In the great scheme of things, not that much, but enough to cause her some serious anguish*).

The police officer spent the next 10 minutes rolling his eyes as he contemplated the paperwork he would have to do.

I tried to cheer him up by telling him that he had personally successfully detected two crimes.

I don't think it worked . . .

🚐 BREATHLESS

The first of my two nights wasn't too bad, I didn't have to wait too long for the ambulances to turn up.

Shame about the second night . . .

My first call was to a 71-year-old female with 'Difficulty in breathing'.

I turned up, and was met by loads of small children. Making my way to the patient, she was using her own home medication to try and ease her asthma.

It wasn't working.

A quick check of her oxygen levels showed 71%. It should be above 95%—anything below 85% makes me rather worried. You might guess that 71% really put the wind up me.

I spoke to the son while preparing my treatment. He'd obviously seen this before, as he gave as good a description of the patient and her problems as I would have expected from a medical professional. The patient had been in intensive care twice for her asthma. If an asthmatic ever ends up in ITU, then it shows how rapidly the patient's condition can deteriorate. At the very least, it makes me rather nervous that the patient will 'go off on me', and suddenly it turns into a respiratory arrest.

The medication was given to the patient, salbutamol—a nebulised drug administered straight into the lungs in the form of a gas. I was also giving her a large amount of pure oxygen in an effort to raise her blood oxygen levels.

Then I turned around and nearly fell over three rows of seven children, quietly sitting cross legged and staring up at me with big brown eyes.

'Don't mind them', said the patient's son, 'It's Eid, so the whole family are celebrating'.

'She', he said indicating the patient, 'has 21 grandchildren'.

I nearly suggested that this might be why she was breathless . . .

So now it was time to wait for the ambulance to take this very sick patient out of my responsibility and off to the hospital. I could see her getting more and more tired, although her oxygen levels were more normal (if only because I was blasting plenty of oxygen down her face-mask).

'Would you please leave the room', asked her

son after talking to the patient, 'she needs to use the commode'.

Now, ask any medical professional when is the most dangerous time for your patient, and I would think that 99% of them would say that it's when they go to the toilet.

'Hmmm . . . alright', I said, 'but someone stays with her'.

I was standing right outside the room, waiting for a shout for help and then for me to bound into the room to resuscitate her in front of 21 small children.

Luckily for all involved she survived her encounter with the commode and we settled down to wait again.

While I was waiting, I was constantly reassessing the patient. I really wasn't happy to have her waiting so long because while my treatment was improving her condition somewhat, she needed better care than I could give.

The son offered me a cup of tea.

He knew how serious it was. He knew that the ambulances in the area were probably picking up drunks, and yet he understood my apologies and offered me a cup of tea.

Thankfully, the ambulance arrived and because of my earlier treatment, the patient had become a little more stable. She still needed urgent hospital care, but I wasn't worried that she would die on the back of the ambulance.

It had taken 45 minutes to get an ambulance to the patient. Sometimes I like it that when I'm on the FRU when I can get to a patient in time to actually make a difference.

I also love the drugs I carry—I don't need to use

them much, but when I need them, they really do come in handy.

I hope everything turned out alright, because, as I followed the crew and the patient out to the ambulance, the son shook my hand and said, 'Thank you'.

. . . Waiting 45 minutes for his critically ill mum to get a proper ambulance, and still he thanked me.

SOFT, WET SNOOKER BALL

The first job of the morning has stayed with me for the rest of the day
—*Warning: not for the faint of heart*—
I was sent to a 'Male, 59, fitting—locked in empty bathroom'. I got there quickly, within 8 minutes, so already it was a 'successful' job.

As the person who met me opened the door to the flat I was overwhelmed with an intense and incredibly disgusting smell. At first I thought that it was the person opening the door (he was rather dishevelled and I've smelt breath that bad before), but no, the smell got stronger as I entered the flat.

There were four people there, all of them looked like the man who opened the door, and the state of the flat made me think that everyone in there was an alcoholic.

Sitting, or rather, propped up on the sofa was the man who had been fitting. His friends had managed to undo the door to the bathroom, and had manhandled him into the living room.

'He's been drinking—we were both drinking heavily yesterday', I was told.

'Fair enough', I said, 'Is he epileptic, or does he have alcoholic fits?'

'Both, I think', replied his friend.

Then I looked down.

Something the size of a snooker ball had rolled down the inside of his jeans and was sitting in front of him. It was brown, it was wet, and was rather horrible looking.

A pile of poo . . . his poo. A poo done after a night of heavy drinking.

Suddenly I realised where the smell was coming from . . .

I'm sure that most people realise that after a night on the town, the first poo you do can stink to high heaven. This was that epic poo. I imagine that there was a lot more of it smeared over the inside of his jeans. This is the sort of poo that would issue forth from the arse of Satan himself. It was the sort of poo that shouldn't be flushed away, but instead sealed in a barrel and buried in a place that has lots of warning signs pinned to the barbed wire fence surrounding it.

It really did smell that bad.

His friend (who actually didn't know him that well), picked up the poo with a bit of newspaper and ran it into the toilet.

I could hear him gagging from his new-found proximity to the toxic poo. When he came back into the room his face was an interesting shade of pale green, and there was a thin film of sweat upon his brow.

I treated the patient—actually quite a simple job. Then the ambulance crew turned up, and I pointed out that the patient's shoe was covered in his own sticky poo.

Carrying the patient down the stairs, the poo managed to get transferred from the shoe onto the shirt of one of the crew. He wasn't happy.

I stopped myself from laughing . . .

. . . *almost*.

The only problem is that I can still, several hours later, smell the rank stench of that demonic poo from hell. Actually, I can still taste the poo in the air.

I almost feel sorry for the nurses at the hospital . . .

THE HUMANITY OF BYSTANDERS

Well that's the last time I say that I haven't had an interesting job all shift . . .

My final job of the day was to a 'Collapsed male in the street'. Unfortunately, Control were having a bit of a computer failure, so the job was given to me the 'old fashioned' way, by someone at Control telling me where to go.

'Collapsed in the street . . . he'll be drunk then', I joked.

No matter, I still raced to the scene as quickly as possible (I've mentioned this before, that what I get called for, and what is actually wrong with the patient are often two very different things—so I always try to get to the job as quickly as possible).

The location wasn't exact, so I spent a bit longer than I would have liked peering down dark streets, looking for a man collapsed on the ground. Some people driving towards me told me that the patient was a bit further down the road.

My heart sank when I saw a huge crowd of people standing around a man lying flat on his

288

back. My heart sank even more when I saw a man doing CPR on the patient.

I jumped out of my car, grabbed my bag and trauma shears and started cutting the patient's clothes off. A quick look at his face, and I didn't hold much hope for him.

'He was jogging, and just collapsed', said one of the men who had been performing CPR, 'he hit his head, we've been doing CPR at 100 compressions a minute'.

'Are you medically trained?', I asked.

'No', he replied, 'I'm a teacher, but I've done a first-aid course'.

'Well', I said, after glancing at the monitor, and noting that there was no activity in the heart at all, 'You were doing really good CPR, so you have given him the best chance he has for survival'.

I just wanted them to know that they were doing the right thing. I knew the patient had pretty much no chance of surviving this event, but that these strangers were trying their best renewed a bit of my faith in human nature.

The ambulance arrived only a few moments after I did, and as I looked at the driver, I could see by the expression on his face that he also realised how serious the situation was.

There was no time for any playing around, so we loaded the patient on the back of the ambulance, and took off for the hospital. I was 'bagging' the patient, while the ambulance attendant was continuing the CPR.

We arrived at the hospital, but there was nothing that they could do.

As he was out jogging, he didn't have any identification at all. We had also taken him to a different hospital than would be expected—it was not the closest hospital by distance, but it was the hospital that we could get to the quickest.

. . . So somewhere, there was probably a family wondering why their husband, or their father, or their brother, or their lover had not come home. They'll ring the local hospital, and they won't have heard of him, and it will only be when they go to the police that they will find out the truth.

I'm also aware that the bystanders who were doing CPR would probably have this event haunting them—I deal with sudden death a lot, but for these people, it was probably the first time they ever had someone die in front of them. I wish there was some way that I could have stayed and made sure that they were alright, and that I was proud of them and that they should be happy that they did the best that they could.

So, a traumatic event for everyone except for us ambulance and hospital staff. And to think that people ask us how we deal with jobs like this . . .

We later found out who he was. Seems like he was a really nice man, which makes his sudden death all the more sad. His family only found out after they went to the police when he didn't return home.

🚑 CRYING

'Two-month-old child—Not waking up'.

'Shit!', I thought (*actually I may have said it*).

'Not waking up' could mean that the child was dead. There was something about the way the job was written up on the terminal screen that made me fear the worst.

I raced around there, brakepads burning and swearing loudly at bus drivers who thought that it might be a good idea to pull out in front of me.

Two minutes thirty seconds later I screeched to a halt outside the house, bounding from the car, grabbing my kit and running into the house.

The baby was crying.

The ambulance crew turned up about 30 seconds later.

I was smiling, the crew were smiling, the mother was smiling. The only person not smiling was the crying baby.

But I was happy at that.

I like children who cry when they see me, it normally means that they aren't seriously ill. It's the quiet ones you have to watch out for.

🚑 NIGHT NUMBER ONE

Bit of a busy night, partly I think due to the frost on the roads. I know that I was not able to drive too fast, as I was occasionally fishtailing across the road. The first job, aptly enough, was a man who had driven his car into a bus. The car was an utter mess, and I would have wanted to immobilise him in the car and have the fire service cut him out. I say *would have wanted* because once the crash was over, he'd run off . . .

So I'm guessing that the car was either stolen, or more likely he just didn't have any insurance, road tax or a driving licence.

A couple of 'nothing' jobs, then another car accident. Some bright spark had decided to borrow his friend's car, and then lose control of it on our main 'A' road. The car, yet again was a write-off, and the driver kept telling me that he was going to 'get done', because he didn't have any insurance . . . or a driving licence.

Can you see a pattern in the drivers from my area?

I then had to go to a 13-year-old child with a progressive and ultimately fatal disease. He was having difficulty in breathing because of a chest infection, and when I got there his breathing was incredibly irregular, and his oxygen levels were only 67% of what they should be. Even with highflow oxygen his oxygen levels were only just adequate.

There was a bit of worry about what I was going to do if he stopped breathing, as he had a 'Do not resuscitate' order, but it was a year out of date.

Thankfully it never came to it, and I was very happy when the crew arrived to take the child to hospital.

My final job was a bit of a nasty one. A young man (a cleaner) was found not breathing in a local supermarket. The call woke me from a light sleep and, as I mentioned, I couldn't drive too quickly to the call. I got there as the ambulance crew arrived, and we were led through the warren of the supermarket by the cleaning supervisor.

The patient was large, covered in blood and vomit, and was not breathing. We attached our heart monitor and it showed no activity in the heart at all. In the process of doing CPR, everything got covered in bloody vomit. As I type this, my jacket is in a plastic bag, waiting to be taken home and washed.

We got him to hospital, but they were unable to save him.

Once more it was a patient who no-one seemed to know (no-one there knew his name, although they had been working with him for a couple of days), and I don't think he had any identification on him.

A tricky job for the police.

A busy night, but as my mum would say, 'At least it made the time go fast'.

MONKEY BALLS, LOSS OF . . .

It is, to put it bluntly, cold enough to freeze the balls off a brass monkey, which is *really* cold.

No matter, it keeps the drunks off the street . . . well, it *mainly* keeps the drunks off the street . . .

I got sent to a '50-year-old man, fallen in street. Blood from ear'. The location was given as 'Outside Red Lion Public House'. I could guess what had happened.

I pulled up, leaving the headlights pointed at the patient, lying on the ground, covered by a blanket borrowed from the pub.

Surrounding him were:

A lot of police (about five or six officers).

Two sons, both of which were crying and worrying about their dad dying.

Some bystanders, most of them had come from the pub, and . . .

One off-duty fireman, who was clutching the patient's hand.

'Fair enough', I thought, 'best get to work'.

The lighting in the street was bad, but my headlights and some police torches made it a little better. The patient had been celebrating in the pub and had tripped over a kerb while trying to walk home. He had possibly been knocked out, and there was some blood coming out of his left ear.

The first thing that you think of when someone who has fallen has blood coming out their ear is that they may have fractured their skull. With a fractured skull you will sometimes get cerebrospinal fluid coming from their ear (cerebrospinal fluid is the liquid that your brain and spinal column float in, and should not be outside the body at all).

The standard test is that blood and CS fluid don't mix, so you'll see yellow streaks in the blood. Given the poor light it was hard to see, so I fell back on an old trick. You stick your (gloved) finger in the blood and if there is CS fluid in it, the blood will feel 'slick'.

The side-effect is that your gloves get covered in blood. It was cold. I wanted to wipe my nose. My gloves were right out, and I wouldn't like to wipe my nose on the cuff of my jacket because it's a disgusting thing to do, and also (mainly) because my jacket is horribly unclean.

The patient also had a large swelling on the back of his head and, because of the way that he had fallen, I couldn't rule out an injury to his neck. In a perfect world I would have liked to have put a cervical collar on him to immobilise his neck, but this is far from a perfect world. A cervical collar only really immobilises a patient if they want to be immobilised, in a drunken or combative patient this will often make them thrash around trying to get it off. So, often a better course of action is to tell them to lie nice and still and leave the collar off until you need to move them.

The off-duty fireman had obviously had a bit of first-aid training, because he was keeping the patient constantly talking. This was fine, as it meant I didn't have to talk to the patient too much, apart from assessing him, and getting his details.

The crowd were pretty well-behaved; I kept hearing one of them moaning that the disabled ramp to the kerb was the reason behind the fall, and that they were 'bloody dangerous'. I didn't want to mention that walking while drunk was perhaps more of a contributing factor . . .

I threw another blanket over the patient because there was little else I could do until the ambulance turned up. Unfortunately, I'd been waiting a long time for ambulances all night, and I suspected that this would be the same.

My nose still threatened to drip on the patient.

Suddenly behind me was a flash of a high-visibility jacket, 'Excellent', I thought, 'the ambulance has turned up'.

But, no, it was one of our duty managers come to see how I was doing. They knew the ambulance would be some time, and wanted to make sure I was alright.

'Ah', he said, 'I can see you have everything under control', and left.

He could have wiped my nose for me . . .

By now I was losing sensation in various small, but important bits of my anatomy. I looked at my watch and saw that I'd been with the patient for over 30 minutes. I was cold, but at least I wasn't lying on the cold wet floor.

Finally the ambulance arrived; they had travelled from out of their area to attend this call, and I was very grateful for them turning up when they did. We put the collar on the patient, strapped him to a stretcher and loaded him into the back of the ambulance where it was much warmer, and I could remove my gloves and wipe my nose.

Can you see what was uppermost on my mind?

The patient was swiftly taken to hospital, and as I prepared to face the crowd of people and explain exactly why the ambulance took so long to arrive, I was instead mobbed by people who wanted to shake my hand and thank me. None of them were bothered by the 40 minutes it had taken the ambulance took to arrive, and they were actually happy that we had done our jobs, accepting that as it was a Friday night we might be a bit busy.

It was only later that I found out that there had been another shooting in the area (some drunk men had been apparently been thrown out of a pub, they then returned and fired a pistol through the pub windows, hitting a barman).

🚑 SICKLE CELL

I'd just done a job with a lovely patient suffering from a sickle cell crisis, but I was shocked when I heard from another crew how the hospital chose to treat her.

This post is one that I've been thinking about writing for at least a year, but I've always been a bit shy of writing it because it touches on possible racism. Just remember, I hate everyone, not just one type of person.

Sickle cell disease is a horrible illness; it results in massive pain, and because of the blood cells 'clumping' it can cause stroke, blindness, kidney failure, heart attacks and numerous other complications. The pain these patients feel is unbelievable.

The thing is, most of these patients are black.

Here is the problem that I have. There are a number of sufferers who are banned from certain emergency departments. There are legal orders that say a patient should not go to a specific A&E when they get a crisis. It's normally because the patient has caused trouble while waiting to be treated; I was an A&E nurse in North London for long enough to realise that some sickle cell disease patients are not saints, but . . .

In my personal experience, sickle cell disease patients are the only patients who get banned from departments. Drunks can be much more violent, yet they never seem to get banned. Some patients are 'Frequent flyers': they attend every day, use up more time and resources than those with sickle cell disease, yet they never seem to get banned. I've also personally witnessed nurses being hit, yet the patient still receives treatment, and is not banned.

While I understand that sickle cell disease patients can be demanding, they are in a huge amount of pain. Some are indeed opioid addicts, but my thoughts on the matter are that it isn't hurting me to give them painkillers, and that the stresses of withdrawal can cause a sickling crisis. However, it does seem that sickle cell patients are being discriminated against.

This affects the ambulance service in the following way: we might pick up a patient 200 yards from the local hospital, he has chest pain, and is in a lot of general all-over pain. If he is banned from that local hospital, we might have to travel miles to get him to a hospital that will accept him. If he has a heart attack or stroke in the back of the ambulance, is it our fault for bypassing a nearby hospital?

These patients often have a 'treatment protocol' at their hospital—this states the type of pain relief that they get, and who should be contacted to continue their treatment. These patients are often concerned that if they are not taken to their specialist centre (always miles away . . .) then the hospital that we do take them to will not have their treatment protocol.

Also, will we be called more because we are now carrying morphine and will maybe give it to patients, when their personalised treatment protocol states that they shouldn't have morphine at all?

In my opinion, sickle cell disease patients are treated poorly in A&E departments, and I don't think that it can be just that they are 'demanding' for their pain relief, or that they are personally 'annoying'. While a lot of these patients can be annoying, I think it's only because they are treated poorly to start with.

Disclaimer—I used to work in an A&E department with a huge population of sickle cell disease patients.

🚑 IQ TEST

General practitioners (family doctors) are supposed to be intelligent . . . right?

So here is a question for you all, answers to the usual address on the back of a £10 note . . .

An elderly patient enters your surgery. She is asthmatic and is having real trouble in breathing. Do you?

(a) Start treating the asthma attack, giving the correct amount of treatment, then when she doesn't improve, call for an ambulance, keeping the patient on oxygen. You then take her vital signs, and observe her closely until the ambulance arrives. You even manage to phone the hospital to refer her to the correct speciality. Or . . .

(b) Give her the paediatric dose of the medicine (the dose you give to under-12s). When she doesn't get any better, you call an ambulance and sit her (without oxygen) out in the waiting room where her wheezing can entertain the toddlers playing there. You write a letter to the hospital, but as you haven't written any vital signs on it, you can't have even taken her pulse in the first place.

Warning, if you answer (b), you then might have to put up with a slightly miffed FRU person explaining that you might have just been a bit silly . . .

There are a scarily large number of GPs who just cannot deal with anyone who might be seriously ill.

Still that's what the LAS are for, and also why we still rush on blue lights and sirens to patients who are being looked after at their GPs.

I could write an entire book about the silly things I've seen doctors do. But I'm of the opinion that I only ever see the results of poor workmanship. The good GPs must be better able to deal with patients without the need for regular ambulance attendance. The next post provided a balancing experience.

🚑 HOW IT SHOULD BE DONE

It was as if my prayers had been answered, a GP who today managed to balance the poor skills of

299

yesterday's doctor.

I was sent to a 74-year-old male with difficulty in breathing and chest pain. My computer display told that me that the GP was going to remain with the patient.

I got there and was met by an apologetic GP who thought that the patient just had a chest infection, but while she was talking to him, the patient developed a possibly heart-related pain. She had tried treating him herself, but thought that the best thing was for him to have some further tests in hospital.

My assessment and treatment of the patient went without a hitch, and I agreed that although I also thought the pain was a consequence of his chest infection, it would be best for the patient to be assessed in the local A&E department.

As was the case yesterday the ambulance was 40 or more minutes in arriving, so I had a bit of a chat with the GP (who was rather pretty . . .) and the patient (not so pretty). As there was nothing else the doctor could do with this patient, I let her leave the house to see her other patients.

A nice job, made easier by another health-care professional.

Just how it should be.

One day I'll have to start counting the number of good GP experiences along with the number of bad GP experiences just so I can get some empirical evidence to prove that there are plenty of good GPs out there.

I was miles out of my area, but this was not a worry, as the sun was shining, the scenery was pretty (well . . . prettier than Newham, not that that this is difficult) and there was some nice music on the radio.

Then the call came down my terminal. 'Male ?Suspended in car'. I consider it a personal strength that I was thinking 'Excellent! I can use my big trauma shears to break a window'.

I soon reached the car and was dismayed to find the passenger door open, and two bystanders watching the man intently.

'He's breathing', they said.

I tried to hide the disappointment that I wouldn't be smashing any windows.

Checking the patient, who was slumped over the passenger seat drooling like a baby, I immediately thought that it would be one of three things: he was either having a diabetic crisis, had just had a stroke or was just incredibly drunk.

A quick test of his blood sugar showed that he wasn't diabetic, a neurological assessment showed that he probably hadn't had a stroke (he was also younger than me, so a stroke would have been rather surprising). This left the last option . . . he was drunk.

Once more I found myself cursing my own particular disability—that I can't smell alcohol. Thankfully, the ambulance crew turned up and let me know that he did indeed stink of booze.

The crew loaded him onto the ambulance, which was tricky as he could hardly walk, while I turned off the engine to his car, amazed that he had driven as far as he had without crashing into something. He was also lucky he'd stopped when he did, as less than 100 metres away was a main road with a speed limit of 50 m.p.h.

We called the police, who duly arrested him. Meanwhile he kept saying that all he wanted to do was die . . .

. . . I would think that his desire to die would only increase as his hangover hits him in the police cell. I got the impression that the reason he was drunk was because he had had an argument with his family.

Somehow I don't think that getting arrested for drink driving (oh, and his tax disc was out of date as well) will do him any good with his family.

See, I keep telling people that getting pissed solves nothing. But do they listen to me? Do they buggery . . .

I had to make a police statement before going back to work, returning just in time to get called to a Bed and Breakfast where an alcoholic was having a panic attack.

GAH!

40 stone patient.
On the floor.
3 hours on scene.
Tears, swearing, pain and blood.
Up to nine staff on scene at once.
I am f*****g knackered. Maybe a more detailed post tomorrow, maybe not.
Gah . . .

I never did write a longer post about that job. So now is my chance.

The patient weighed around 42 stone and was stuck on the toilet—this is when I arrived. In an effort to get her up she managed to slip onto the floor, which was better for her as the blood flow to her legs returned. An ambulance crew turned up and we had a little conference about what to do. The fire service were asked to attend, but they decided not to, as it's now against their policy to help us lift heavy patients. By now the family were starting to get angry at the patient.

Our Control suggested a 'Mangar Elk' which is a lifting aid that uses compressed air to raise patients off the floor. So along came a Duty Officer and a Training Officer with the bit of kit and the expertise to use it.

Our Complex boss turned up and fed the patient some chocolate biscuits—we looked at him in a most stern manner and he left.

We phoned the local hospital to pre-warn them and they tried to refuse the patient. Our Duty Officer had a chat with them on the phone and after much to'ing and fro'ing they agreed to accept them.

The patient was frightened about leaving the house. The family were getting more and more annoyed at the patient . . .

. . . Then the patient's drunk partner turned up.

After several attempts we managed to get the patient out the house and into the ambulance.

Just.

🚑 TICKETS

I've checked with my sources, and the story is true.

At Poplar ambulance station there is no room to

park. The station itself is tiny, barely bigger than a portacabin. There is a big metal fence and electric gate around it. There is minimal parking.

So the ambulances park out on the street—if they didn't then every emergency call would be delayed by minutes as the crews wait for the gate to open and then manoeuvre the ambulances out. This would be very bad for the patients (and more importantly, extremely bad for our ORCON times).

There is nowhere else to park.

So . . . a couple of days ago the ambulances all got parking tickets.

Apparently there is a man who lives in one of the nearby tower blocks who keeps complaining because his daughter nearly had an accident pulling out of the turning.

So a nice man from the council (or a parking warden) came around and put tickets on the ambulances. In his defence he did try to not ticket them by telling the crews to drive around the block . . .

The ambulance crews find this all very amusing.

(*We are, by our driving exemptions, allowed to park where we like as long as it's not 'dangerous'; we are guessing that this man has complained so much the council has been spurred into action.*)

It's not the first time this has happened, and it won't be the last. I feel sorry for the warden who has to give the tickets—it can't do much for the reputation of ticket wardens to be seen sticking one on an ambulance.

HEALTH FORECASTS

Did you know that the Meteorological Office offers 'health forecasts'? We got a memo from them (via our office) about a predicted increase in paediatric respiratory infections.

No kidding! For 2 days all I attended were patients with chest infections.

Then on Friday all but two of my 13 calls were faints, or epileptic fits. I'm left wondering if it is something in the weather that caused that little spike.

Oh, I also attended three schools on Friday (one epileptic and two fainters), while normally I wouldn't see that many schools in on month.

A strange day.

Is it any wonder us ambulance folk are a superstitious lot?

WE SOMETIMES DO GOOD WORK

We deal with a lot of crap jobs on a day to day basis, but when we are really needed I think we do a bloody good job.

One of the people injured in the London bombings is getting married this weekend.

The thing that gets me is this quote.

'As well as losing both feet in the bombing, Ms Hicks lost 75 per cent of her blood and her heart stopped twice on the way to the hospital.'

That means that an ambulance crew successfully resuscitated her twice—long enough to get her to hospital—and that because of that unnamed crew she is now alive and getting married. It's stories like that which makes me happy to do the work that I do; sometimes we can make a difference.

I was talking about this story with one of my station-mates. He'd seen the report on the television and was astounded—not only because he had been the one to run her into hospital, but also because he thought that she would have died. So congratulations to the crew involved, Brian Robinson and Lisa Isaacs—you did us all proud.

R+J = GBH?

'Warning: Assailant may still be on scene, wait for police' had apparently flashed up on my computer screen. Unfortunately, it had done so silently, so the first I saw it I was pulling up outside the house. Luckily, I was pulling up to the house which had a police car outside it.

I entered a house that was full of four generations of Bangladeshi people who were mainly shouting at each other and the two beleaguered police officers. Quite rightly so I thought, as I looked at the 15-year-old boy I had been called to treat. He had been hit around the head with a metal bar. Thankfully, his injuries were fairly minor, although there was a possibility that he had broken his elbow.

Unfortunately, this was one of those nights where ambulances were a bit thin on the ground, so I was waiting for some time. At least this meant I was able to get the reasoning behind what had been happening.

There were two families, one with a daughter, the other had a son (my patient). He had

306

apparently offered her a place to sleep after she had been in an argument with her family. This had then turned into a feud that had dragged on via school bullying. The police had just told everyone present that they would be going around the other family's house to arrest people when the father of this family turned up.

To say there was a lot of shouting would be an understatement. There was also a procession of stern young men in the garden having a bit of a war council, mobile phones clamped to ears as they called in reinforcements. The atmosphere was getting a trifle warm for my liking.

Luckily the police were able to calm the situation down somewhat, a bit tricky when the father was shouting about how he was going to burn the other family's house down if they didn't do anything. Meanwhile, large numbers of youths were appearing and disappearing into the night. I thought that there was a real chance of things turning nasty.

'Sir', said one of the policemen, 'I don't wish to insult, or cause offence, but normally with this kind of trouble it is one cultural group against another, but in this case both parties are Bangladeshi. Could you explain that to me?'

One of the calmer young men replied, 'That's how it *used* to be, now everyone is fighting everyone else, and race doesn't matter'.

By now I had the real impression of angry villagers with pitchforks and flaming torches gathering. Thankfully, I was rescued by both police backup and an ambulance to take the injured party away to hospital.

'Control', I called up on my radio, 'Just to make

you aware, if there are any assaults in this part of my patch, don't let crews go in without police escort, because it might kick off big time'.

'Roger that EC50, I'll make a note'.

I don't think that there was any trouble that night, but it is a little hard to lynch someone if you (or they) have been arrested . . .

THE FRIDAY BEFORE CHRISTMAS

It's the busiest night of the year for us, as everyone goes out and gets drunk at their work Christmas party. I don't know what's going on at the moment, but it's barely 21:00 and already we are at 3 500 or more calls.

We normally do 3 500 calls in a day, so how many more will we squeeze in over the next 3 hours?

My first job was to an alcoholic having had a fit. A common symptom of being an alcoholic is having fits. I'd say that of the two types of fits that we go to, I tend to see more alcoholic fits than epileptic fits. I don't have any numbers to prove it, but it just seems right in my experience.

This job was typical. I had to step over the detritus on the carpet, the packets of tobacco, the trainers and the half-eaten takeaway container. I saw my patient sitting on a chair, being sick. He was vomiting directly onto the living room floor, his wife didn't see fit to put a bucket under the stream of vomit.

Lovely.

Like a lot of our regular alcoholic customers, he was topless, while his tracksuit bottoms were stained with . . . well I wouldn't like to guess, but they were stained with something. Homemade tattoos covered his chest, arms and hands, and in between bouts of vomiting he would continue making a roll-up cigarette.

'Can I turn the living room light on?', I asked the wife.

'Don't work', she said back to me in a voice that I guessed had been arguing with her husband just before I'd arrived.

I guessed this because she then started arguing with him again.

While the living room had a nice stereo, a reasonable television (satellite included) and a gaming console, they didn't have a light bulb.

He didn't want to go to hospital, but I always think of the potential headlines in the paper the next day 'Ambulance leave patient to die', so the crew and I persuaded him to go to hospital for a 'check-up'.

You know why? No one ever lost their job by taking a patient to hospital.

'I don't want to waste their time', he mumbled, 'I'm just an alcoholic'.

'It's alright mate', I'd reply, 'We look after everyone, even alcoholics'.

There were around 5200 jobs that day up to midnight and over 1000 calls before 3 a.m. the following morning.

PANIC ON THE STREETS OF LONDON

When I'm at a 'job' I don't panic, it's part of my job description to keep control of a situation and to stop other people from running around like headless chickens. Sometimes I will have to be forceful, or act quickly, but I *never* panic.

I got a job, '14-month-child, floppy and lifeless'.

'Fuck', I thought.

It was in a part of my patch I'm not very familiar with—new buildings on the Isle of Dogs. The address was given as 'Flat 1, Rose House, Starling Road'.

This is obviously not the address I was given, I do respect patient confidentiality after all.

I rushed to Starling Road, a new estate with loads of buildings, none of which seemed to be marked.

'Fuck', I thought.

If a child is floppy or lifeless, then the chances are it is either *very* ill, or is dead.

I sped up and down the road. I spotted some of the names of the flats in tiny writing, on little blue plaques, many of them pointing away from the road. My pulse started to race. It had taken me 4 minutes to reach the area, but how much longer would it take me to locate the potentially very sick child?

I found 'Lilac House', 'Lily House' and 'Tulip House', but I couldn't find 'Rose House'.

Now I was starting to panic. Was I being stupid? Had I driven past it? Was the baby dead, and if it was, was it because I couldn't find the fucking house?

I could feel the sweat soaking my back, without being able to get to the patient there was nothing I could do. I cursed the council, the builders, the architects—everyone who had thought that putting pretty but bloody useless signs on the buildings was a good idea.

I got Control to ring the parents back, the mother came out to meet me. 'Rose House' was behind another block of flats, behind a road barrier. The name plaque had text around an inch high, pointing away from the road.

Luckily the baby only had a runny nose.

I hated it though, the utter feeling of helplessness that comes with being unable to find a patient—the sweating, the raised pulse and the vaguely sick feeling in the bottom of the stomach as you race up and down a street in the dark trying to find the right location.

Please. If any architects, builders, council planners or sign writers read this, make the signs bigger. Make them so I can read them at night. Make them so that if it is *your* relative that is critically ill, I can find them before it is too late.

I got a comment from an architect explaining that they get no say in the marking of the houses they design—so I'd like to apologise for including them in this rant. However, can I then take the opportunity to shout at architects who think that spiral staircases are a good idea? If you ever try to carry a patient down a spiral staircase you'll find that it's bloody hard work, if not impossible.

🚑 RANT ALERT! RANT ALERT!

The past couple of nights I've gone to calls that I've wanted to grab some parents and shake some common sense into them. Instead, I have to be polite, if only for the quiet life.

Apologies—Judgemental post ahoy!

'Madam', I hear myself say, 'the reason that your

four children have asthma may well have something to do with the four packs of cigarettes I see sitting on the sofa. When you were at the antenatal classes, and they told you the effects of smoking on your children, did you think that they just liked to hear the sound of their own voices? Or, did you in an uncharacteristic spark of intelligence, think that they may just be the agents of some vast conspiracy financed by the companies who make nicotine patches?'

'You might also consider that the reason all your children have runny noses, is because smoking makes them less likely to fight off respiratory infections. You might not know this, but asthma kills people, and that includes children. You are condemning them to a shortened life of ill health and hospital visits, all so that you can feed your oral fixation.'

To other parents I might say . . .

'So, when you got an electric shock from the uninsulated wire poking from that hole in the wall, you didn't think of . . . I don't know . . . let's say . . . protecting your children by having it fixed? Sure, it might cost you a bit of money, but at least your toddler wouldn't now be in hospital to make sure that being electrocuted by mains electricity didn't do any permanent harm'.

'I like that toy', I'd say to another mother of two, 'I particularly like the little bite-sized bits of plastic that are strewn over the floor. Yes, I understand that your oldest child is a mite untidy . . . but when your 18-month-old is choking to death on a toy soldier, some might consider it too late to tidy up. I know it's hard to teach 6-year-olds to clean up after themselves, especially one who seems to be happier peeling your wallpaper off the wall while you shout at him to 'stop fuckin' doin' that!'. Perhaps you might try a different approach? In answer to your question, no you can't smoke in the back of the ambulance'.

To one angry parent I might say . . .

'So your baby stopped breathing for 5 minutes . . . and I took over half an hour to come? Well, I'd like to show you the time you called, and how it took me only 2 minutes to get here, but I think the computer display in my car might confuse you. Besides, I'm not delivering your pizza, you don't get your money back if I'm longer than 30 minutes. Still, back to the baby—she's breathing alright now, perhaps I could interest you in employment in the ambulance service, as you seem to have a Christ-like ability to get children breathing again. Oh, sorry, baby is a 'he' not a 'she'? Sorry, I was confused at the two hoop earrings, the three necklaces, and the rings—all at under 6 months. Why stop there? Maybe they would like their belly button pierced as well? Still I suppose Shayne is a manly name—funny way of spelling it though. Never mind, we're off to hospital now, don't forget your fags'.

And don't forget those who may have strange priorities . . .

'JESUS CHRIST! Aren't the 6-foot Santas and inflatable snowmen supposed to be outside the house? I thought I was going to get mugged by a madman in red. Nice television though, if you could just turn the volume down a little so I can hear what you are saying to me. Yes Tyler is an adorable 8-year-old, even if he did injure himself smashing his neighbour's windows. Why, might I

313

ask are his hands that colour? Ah, how silly of me, paint from his self expression in the fine art of graffiti. Did you consider a taxi to take you the 400 yards to hospital? You can't afford one? Ever think of selling the TV? Or maybe the Santa? Yes, yes, you can bring your cigarettes'.

And breathe . . . and relax . . .

It was supposed to end at the first paragraph, but I just kept rolling . . . Oops.

I'm not normally so hateful . . . Honest.

🚐 WHY I HATE SMOKING PARENTS

This followed a bit of a naughty post about mothers smoking in front of their children—while pregnant. In it I try to explain why I'm a bit of a health Nazi about smoking in front of children.

From my nursing days—a reason why I hate people who smoke around children.

Eight-year-old girls don't look like they are sleeping when they are dead. At least not after over an hour of trying to save her life from an ultimately fatal asthma attack.

We were all distressed, she had been gasping for breath when the ambulance crew had 'blued' her straight into resus'. Asthma nebulisers hadn't worked, and all anyone could fixate on was her chest desperately trying to pull air into her lungs.

She died a frightening and painful death.

The doctor and I went to tell her parents. They were in the relatives' room, I could barely see them as I walked in—clouds of smoke filled the air.

They cried, of course they cried.

Then they went outside and had a cigarette.

314

Then they came back inside the Resus' room and sat with her body.

The father lit up another cigarette.

This is why I hate asthma; this is why I hate people who smoke when they are pregnant; this is why I hate people who smoke around children. Kill yourself if you want to, but don't kill your kids.

There are jobs that haunt you. This was one of them. Try calming down an 8-year-old girl who is dying in front of you because they can't breathe. Then try and forget about it. I did a cot death once, beside the cot was a full ashtray. Sure, the parents are punished by the death of their child. But it doesn't help the child . . .

. . . As I typed this I realised that I was clenching my teeth.

🚑 CAN'T BE BOTHERED

I've just come from a call to one of my semi-regulars. He's alcoholic, has a stomach ulcer and is as thin as a rake. He is sitting in a filthy kitchen surrounded by empty bottles of cheap booze.

He's 26 years old.

His friend, of the same age, is also an alcoholic. He has pancreatitis.

Asked if they want to try a rehab' programme, I was told that they weren't interested.

I've got to confess, it made me angry. Two lives being washed away with bottles of cheap cider.

'So you want to die?' I asked.

They didn't have an answer.

Now I just want to hit something.

315

Anger for all the usual reasons—that I hate to see people throwing their lives away.

🚐 SPACES

Sleep deprivation does funny things to my mind.

I'm having a bit of an insomnia moment, so I turn on the television and randomly tune it to various stations. I come across the 'extreme sports' channel, and watch a film about skateboarders and parkour runners. As I'm watching them using steps, guard rails, benches, ramps, statues and other street furniture to make their way across town in an interesting way, I start to wonder if they see the city in a different way to the rest of us. Do they see jumps, 'grinds' and the like on an almost unconscious level?

Then I start thinking about how I see the place where I work. I see it on three different levels. I see the streets as a map. Main roads to use in order to get to the different areas of town, the junctions that I always seem to be taking, turning left to get to the police station, turning right to head towards Forest Gate. Turning right here to get to Leyton, or straight on towards Stratford. It's all there in my head in the white and yellow of the A to Z. This is the way I think of Newham as I'm going to a job.

The other way that I think of the streets is as I'm trying to make my way through the traffic. I stop seeing cars and lorries as vehicles. Instead, I'm watching the spaces that they make. I'm watching the patterns they make in the road ahead. I'm unconsciously aware of where the drivers are looking: have they seen me or not? The way the

316

vehicles move is also in my mind. Are they hesitant? If they are then there is a good chance that they will stop suddenly. Are they speeding? In that case they may overtake the car that has seen me and has pulled over. I spend my time seeing, and aiming for the spaces.

Finally, I see Newham in terms of the patients I have treated. Over there was the 34-year-old who dropped dead playing football. Across the road is one of our regulars, a lovely old lady with a list of ailments as long as your arm. That street I'm about to pull into had the drunk who didn't notice that he had a broken hand. Now I'm cruising past the road that a 12-year-old died in. A hundred yards from where I'm eating my McBagel is where the teenager got stabbed after the Notting Hill carnival. Every street has a story, and some memories are always triggered as I drive past them. For me, Newham is full of ghosts.

🚑 HAPPY CHRISTMAS . . .

Just been to a young woman in her late 20s.
Deceased.
Leaves behind two children.
Happy Christmas.

🚑 LEXICON OF THE LAS
(OR WHAT 'PUNTER' MEANS)

999—The number you dial to get the ambulance. Equivalent to the American 911 or European 112.

A&E—'Accident and Emergency', also known as 'Casualty' or 'ER—Emergency Room'. Where we take our patients in an effort to make them feel better.

Alkie—An Alcoholic.

Amber Call—in contrast with a 'Cat A' these are the less serious calls. Stuff like simple accidents, broken legs, epileptic fits.

'Ambo', 'Big White Taxi', 'Motor', 'Truck', 'Drunkmobile', 'Barely working shitheap'—Ambulance

Bent—Wrong, illegal, corrupt, or a derogatory term for a homosexual. Used as . . . 'That car radio is bent', 'That bloke is bent' or 'All the police are bent'. Also used as 'running back bent' meaning going for food/back to station without letting Control know about it.

Bloke, Fella—Male person.

CAC—Central Ambulance Control, full of people who actually take the 999 calls, and others who dispatch us to the jobs. They have air conditioning and don't actually smell the patients that they send us to. Recently renamed to EOC (Emergency Operations Centre).

CAD Number—Computer Aided Dispatch. Each job has its own number refreshed each day, because of this I can tell you that the LAS goes to more than 3500 calls every day.

318

Cat A—A high-priority emergency call. This is the priority that cardiac arrests get, along with chest pains, difficulty in breathing and the like. These are timed with ORCON, which I often rant about . . .

Chav—Like a *scrote*, only with more money.

CPN—Community Psychiatric Nurse, an often useless person who visits people with mental health problems in the community. See previous posts for more information.

ECG (EKG)—An examination of the heart using electrical impulses generated by the heart. If you are in an ambulance and the crew start to look worried at the printout you may be in trouble.

EMT—Emergency Medical Technician.

EC/NE/NW/SE/SW/C—the sectors of the London Ambulance Service; East Central, North East, North West etc. . . .

GBH—Grievous Bodily Harm, an assault that breaks a bone or other serious injury. Someone who is going to bleed over the back of your motor.

GP—Family health provider. We only get to see the crap ones who sit patients having heart attacks out in their waiting room and don't even give them an aspirin.

Green Call—Lowest priority: cut fingers, coughs and runny noses. Often mistaken with Cat As because people who call ambulances for a cough often complain of chest pain and difficulty in breathing.

HEMS—Helicopter Emergency Medical Service, in London the medical helicopter that flies out of the Royal London hospital. Staffed with a doctor and a paramedic they fly out to serious cases. Funded by charity and corporate sponsorship.

IVDU—Someone who injects illegal drugs intravenously, mainly a heroin addict.

LAS—London Ambulance Service, the company I work for, also called 'Da Firm' by those of us on the ground floor. Run by 'Da Boss' Peter Bradley, who is generally well liked by us grunts; he is considered a hell of a lot better than his predecessors.

LOL—Not, as Internet people will tell you, 'Laugh Out Loud', but 'Little Old Lady'; a group of patients who spend half their time throwing themselves on the floor, breaking their bones and having urine infections.

Matern-a-taxi—What an ambulance turns into when transporting a near-term pregnancy who is having contractions every '2 minutes' yet you don't see anything approaching a contraction during the 30-minute journey.

MDT—Mobile Display Terminal; the computer screen installed in the ambulance that, running Windows in-between crashing, gives us the details of jobs.

Native—In East London a person from an ethnic minority, mainly because there are more ethnic minorities than 'white British'. This isn't actually an insult, more a running joke.

NHS—The National Health Service, the 'free at point of access' health-care system of Britain. Paid for by taxes, it is on the point of collapse. Split into a number of 'trusts' which include hospitals, GPs and ambulance services.

NHS Direct—Another telephone advice service, staffed by nurses: they will tell you to call an ambulance for having a cold. Ring 0845 46 47 for 24-hour advice. Often disparagingly called 'NHS Re-Direct'.

Plod, Boys in Blue, Old Bill, Fuzz, Coppers—The police; a bunch of folks we tend to get on well with, especially if they let us off speeding when they find out who we work for.

Popper—Someone who injects drugs subcutaneously; a handful died in Glasgow a little while ago from an infected source, leading to much merriment for the local ambo crews.

Punter—A patient (or 'client' if you want to sound like a twit); from a slang term used by second-hand car salesman, actually meaning a gambler, or one who is about to make a gamble (so, therefore, a stunningly accurate description of our patients).

Purple, Purple Plus—A dead body, the 'plus' indicates a body that has been dead for some time;

often recognisable when you walk in the front door and are hit by the smell.

RTA—Road Traffic Accident, the British version of a MVA. Now called a 'Road Traffic Collision' in an attempt to stop lawyers getting their clients off the hook by telling the court that the police have already called it an 'accident'.

Scrote—An often alcoholic person with more tattoos than teeth, bad hygiene and a poor attitude towards employment. Scrote is also short for scrotum.

TAS—Telephone Advice Service; when someone calls for an ambulance for some minor crap they may sometimes be diverted to the TAS desk at CAC for advice, this saves us going to about 200 calls a day across London.

Tramp juice—Super strength lager or cider, sold cheap. Examples include 'White Lightning' and 'Tennents Super', empty cans of which, when found in the street, signify the less salubrious parts of town.

VF/VT/Asystole/PEA—The beating of the heart is normally 'sinus rhythm' VF/VT/asystole/PEA are the names of heart rhythms that are ultimately fatal. VF (ventricular fibrillation) and VT (ventricular tachycardia) we can 'shock' with a defibrillator to try and restore a normal heartbeat, asystole and PEA (pulseless electrical activity) can't be shocked.

322

Wanker—Technically, someone who masturbates. In reality, a fairly mild insult.

Watersquirters, LFB, Mobile Drip Stands, Trumpton—The fire service; a bunch of part-timers who get to sleep all night as there are very few fires in London and no-one cares if cats get stuck in trees during the night. Unlike in the USA, we are two very separate services.

ACKNOWLEDGEMENTS

On July 22nd 2003 a trainee Emergency Medical Technician by the name of Brian Kellett started writing a blog under the pseudonym 'Tom Reynolds'.

Since then more people have come to know me as Tom Reynolds than as Brian.

The blog this book is based on would have never happened if I had not been inspired by writers such as Diamond Geezer (http://diamondgeezer. blogspot.com), Euan Semple (The Obvious http://theobvious.typepad. com/blog/), Warren Ellis (http://www.warrenellis.com), Pixeldiva (http:// www.pixeldiva.co.uk/), Joey DeVilla (Adventures of Accordion Guy http://accordionguy.blogware.com/blog) and Suw Charman (Chocolate and Vodka http://chocnvodka.blogware.com/blog)

It was Jane Perrone (http://perrone.blogs.com/ horticultural/) a writer for *The Guardian*, who, with one mention, attracted thousands of readers to my site.

Now, a couple of years later my blog has changed my life.

I've met people I'd never have met, and been places and done things that I'd never have considered. Most importantly, I was introduced into the larger community of blog writers, who hail from every walk of life, with every experience under the sun and who let me understand life from a million points of view.

This book is a collection of some of my favourite

posts. If you like them, you'll find more on my blog. I write roughly five times a week, so by the time you read this there will be plenty of new material.

I should also like to thank everyone who has had to work with me in the ambulance service—sometimes knowing full well that I was gathering ideas for the blog. Also thanks to my bosses, who haven't sacked me for blogging about the things we sometimes have to do.

I can't finish this without thanking Pat and Brett, my mum and my brother, without whom I would not be the person I am today.

Keep Safe.

Tom Reynolds (a.k.a Brian Kellett)
http://randomreality.blogware.com/blog/

cox

636
101
366
378
252
1343
65
1059